Surprising, Inspiring Birth

Birth accounts to inform, amuse and reassure

Other books by Sylvie Donna:

Preparing for a Healthy Birth

A 10-step guide to help women prepare for healthy, safe births,
with information not usually available to pregnant women, and birth stories.
Available in British and American editions, with or without references.
Includes a quick-reference glossary of pregnancy terms and a full index.

Better Pregnancy, Better Birth

A week-by-week guide to pregnancy and birth, without birth stories but with
notes and references to academic research, in case you need them.
Includes a quick-reference glossary of pregnancy terms and a full index.

Optimal Birth: What, Why & How

A book for students, midwives and other caregivers
with full notes and references to academic research

All Fresh Heart books are available from Amazon,
the Fresh Heart website or from any good bookstore near you!

Surprising, Inspiring Birth

Birth accounts to inform, amuse and reassure

Introduced and edited by

Sylvie Donna

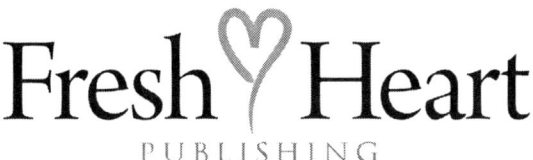

Fresh Heart PUBLISHING

Published in Great Britain in 2010 by
FRESH HEART PUBLISHING
a division of Fresh Heart
PO Box 225, Chester le Street, DH3 9BQ
www.freshheartpublishing.com
www.freshheartpublishing.co.uk

First edition 2010
ISBN: 978 1 906619 12 1

A CIP catalogue record for this publication is available from the British Library

Set in Franklin Gothic
Cover design by Fresh Heart Publishing
Cover photo of one of the fathers whose babies' births are described in this book... you will have to read the book to find out who it is precisely!
Designed and typeset by Fresh Heart Publishing
Printed in the UK by Lightning Source UK Ltd

Disclaimer

While the advice and information contained in this book is believed to be accurate and true at the time of going to press, neither the author nor the publisher can accept any legal responsibility for loss, damage or injury occasioned to any person acting or refraining from action as a result of information contained herein. The advice is intended as a guideline only and should never be used as a replacement for consultation with midwives, doctors or consultants.

Photo © Nina Klose

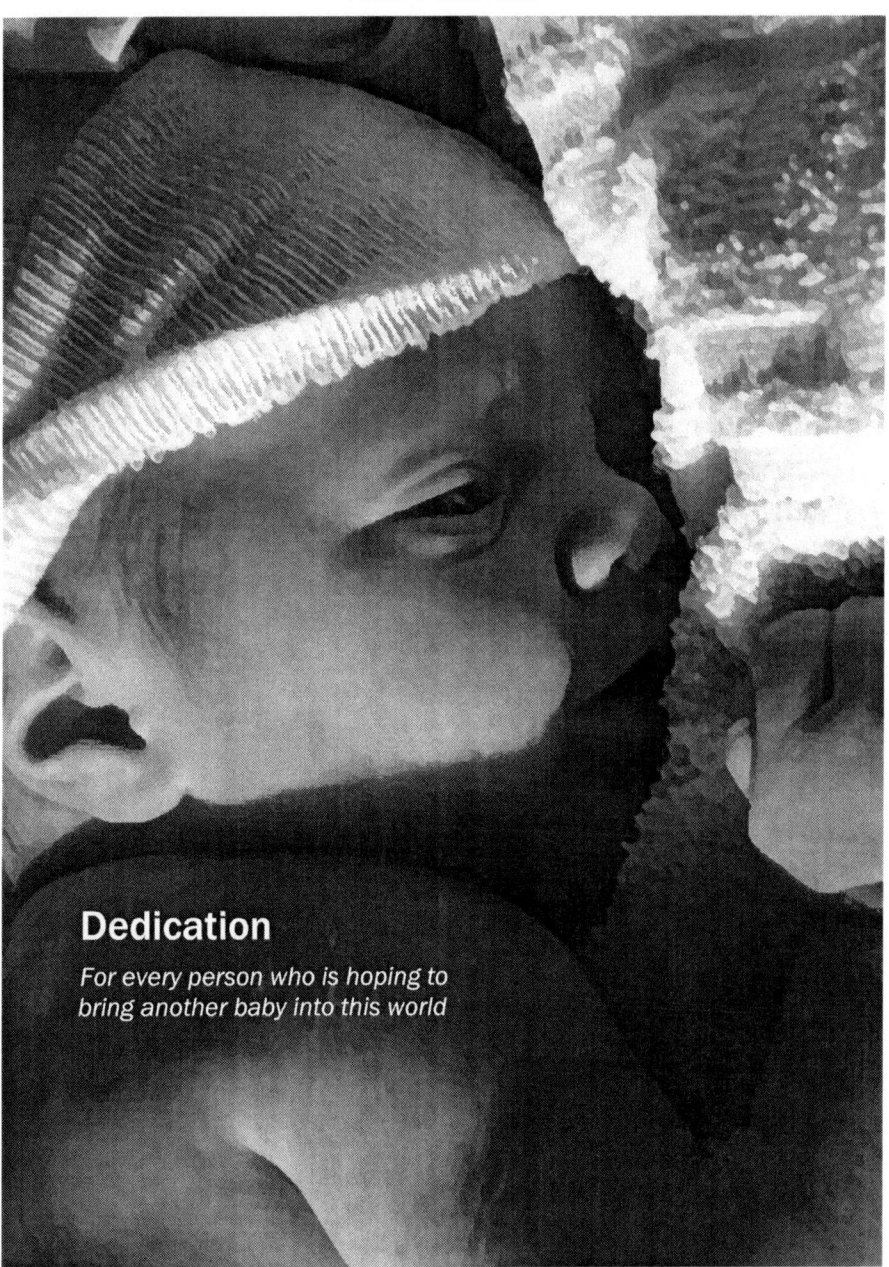

Dedication

*For every person who is hoping to
bring another baby into this world*

A newborn baby

Photo © Nina Klose

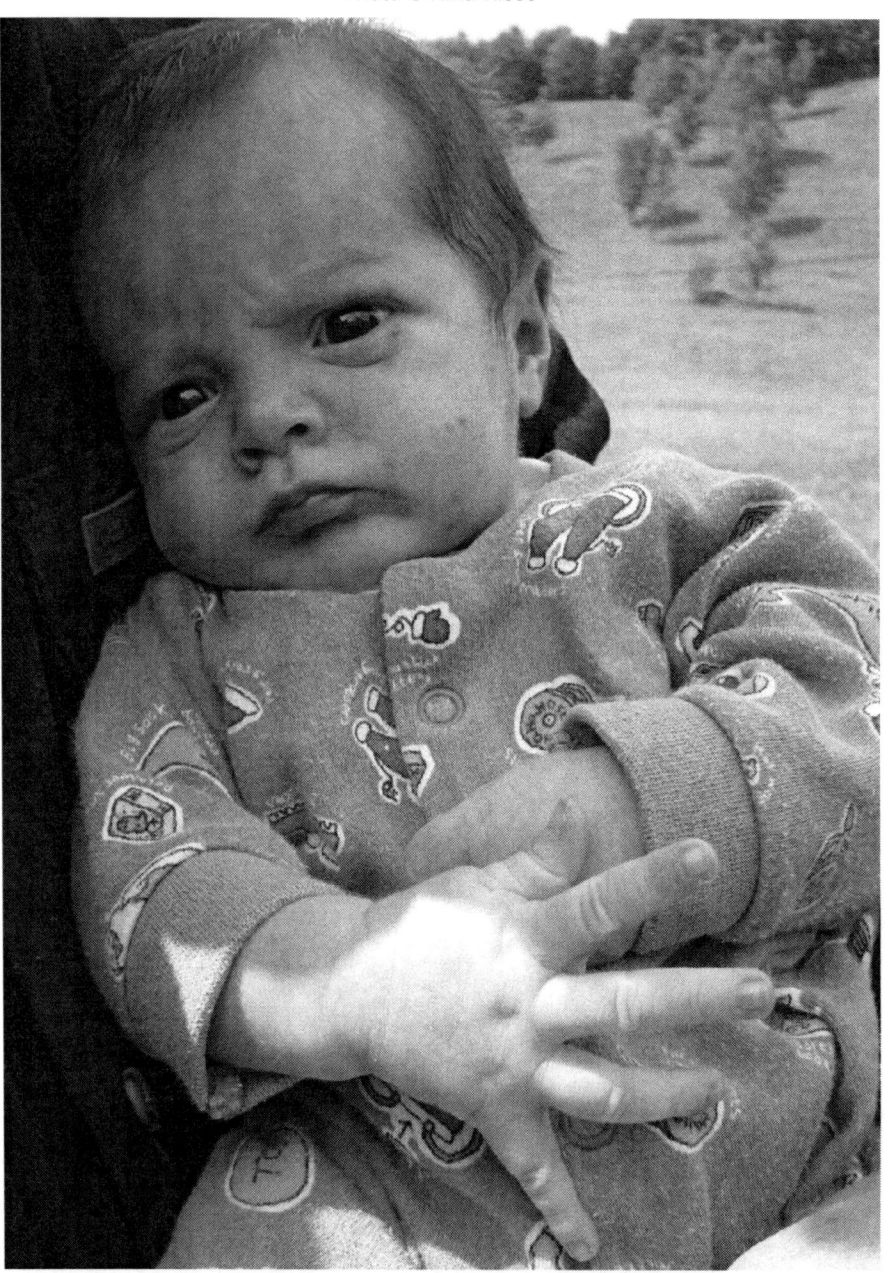

The same baby, a few weeks later...

Contents

Coping with high risk and actual problems... 65

Overcoming bad first experiences... 93

Testing the limits of possibility... 120

Ordinary, extraordinary adjustments... 140

Acknowledgements

While researching the book *Preparing for a Healthy Birth,* which provides information and inspiration for pregnant women, I gathered a great deal of material. It was very difficult to select material for that book and also for this book of birth stories! I based my final decisions on what I felt would be most useful for a pregnant woman and her partner to read.

For the material used in this book, I would like to thank the following:

Phil Anderton, Elaine Batchelor, Sarah Cave, Ruth Clark, Kathryn Clarke, Krisanne Collard, Esther Culpin, Mave Denyer, Beth Dubois, Pauline Farrance, Sarah-Jane Forder, Janet Hanton, Sarah Hobart, Angela Horn, Jennifer Jacoby, Nina Klose, Tanya Kudryashova, Liliana Lammers, Alan Low, Christina Mansi, Ashley Marshall, Steve and Olga Mellor, Michel Odent, Nuala OSullivan, Sue Pakes, Gaia Pollini, Justine Renwick, Jenny Sanderson, Maria Shanahan, Laura Shanley, Debbie Shaw, Gemma Shepherd, Fiona Lucy Stoppard, Rachel Urbach, Ulrike von Moltke, Michael White and Liz Woolley—as well as the women who preferred (or needed) to remain anonymous.

For the use of all the wonderful photographs I would like to thank those same people, as well as Jill Furmanovsky and Colin Smith.

Finally, I would like to thank all the researchers, midwives, obstetricians and other caregivers who have supported me by answering questions or providing information on request. Your support has been invaluable.

The publisher would also like to thank the following for the use of previously published material:
- Shufu no Tomosya for the photograph of Liliana Lammers which was originally published in the Japanese-language magazine *Balloon* (page 104)
- *LLL GB News* for allowing the publication of an adapted, extended version of an account by Sarah Jane-Forder, which appeared in the magazine
- *New Beginnings* for allowing the publication of a longer version of an account by Beth Dubois, which originally appeared in the May/June 2003 issue

The publisher was unable to contact the copyright holder of the photos of Mave Denyer, after repeated attempts.

If any material has accidentally been used without appropriate acknowledgement, or if any details are incorrect, please contact the publisher so that amendments can be made in future editions. Every possible effort has been made to ensure that all details of contributions are correct.

Photo © Colin Smith

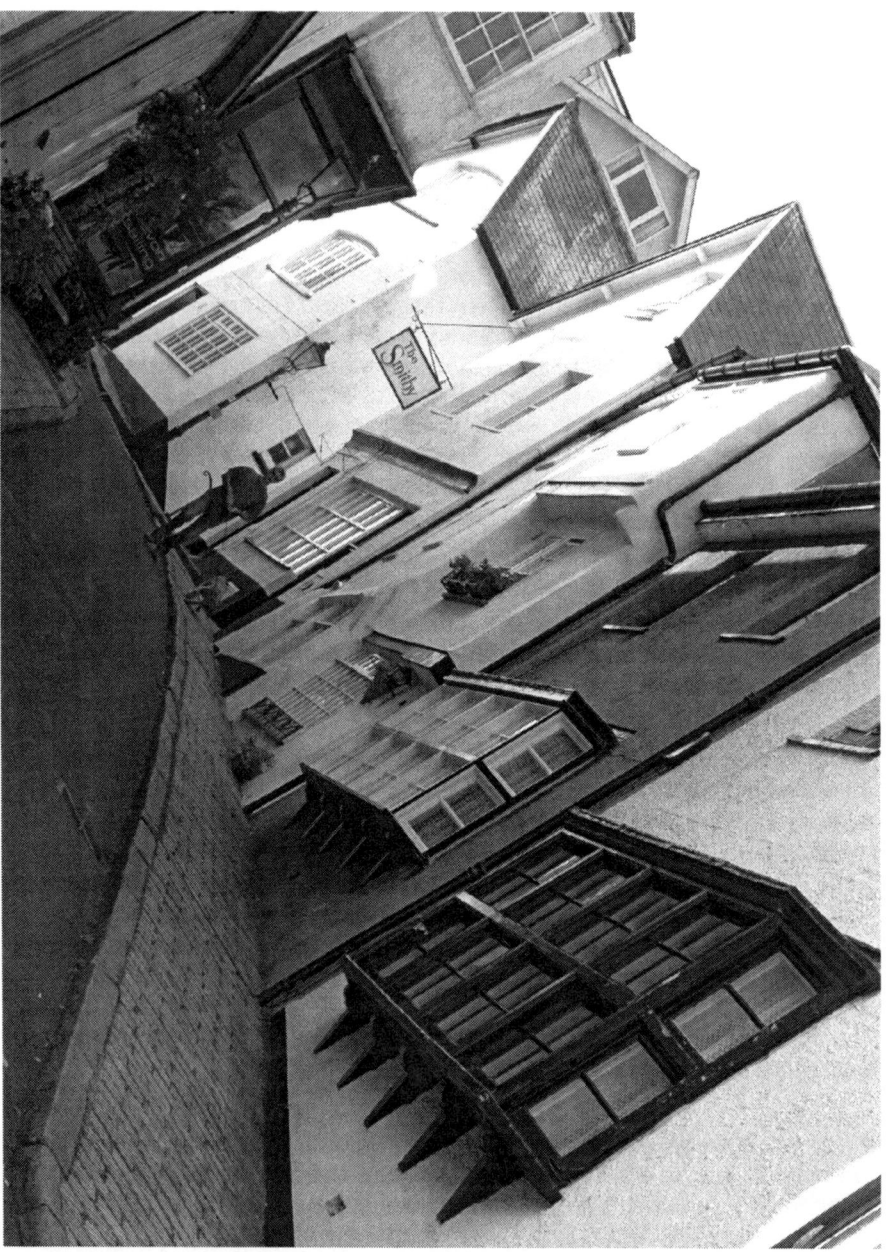

*When you're thinking about getting pregnant—or even worse, when you are!—
the world might suddenly seem to be a very unfamiliar place...*

Introduction:
You mean, you had no drugs?!

This book is mainly about births which took place without any drugs... That doesn't mean there was no pain relief and it also doesn't necessarily mean that the women who gave birth experienced outrageous pain. Some did, some didn't... Some women these days even talk about having orgasmic births!

Whatever sensations women experience while they are in labour and giving birth (whether excruciating or orgasmic), the mums-to-be featured in this book all chose to avoid the use of drugs if at all possible. If this shocks you, consider this email, which I received from a woman who you'll read about soon:

From: Beth Dubois
To: Sylvie Donna
Sent: 29 June, 12:57
Subject: Pain!

Hi Sylvie,
Your book sounds like it will be very encouraging for women. It makes me think of an interesting dream I had some months after the birth. A pregnant woman was telling a group of mothers how she was planning to have an epidural, which she said had been great for her during her first child's birth. When I heard her (despite the incredible birthing experience I'd had), I felt doubt about whether there was really any benefit to experiencing the pain of labour and birth. That night I had a dream in which Valerie, my midwife, was my fitness coach. She was coaching me on some particular physical fitness challenge, like an obstacle course. I had previously not been able to do it at all. Suddenly, now that I had given birth, I was able to fly through the fitness course nearly effortlessly. I was amazed at how what had once seemed nearly impossible was now easy. What I got from this dream was that the experience of giving birth naturally had changed me at a very profound level and was totally worthwhile.

As well as being incredibly empowering, a normal healthy birth without drugs is also much better for you and your future babies. Here's why...
♥ Without any drugs or unnecessary interventions, your labour is likely to proceed much more smoothly. Literally nothing will be disturbing the normal, healthy, hormonal processes. (If your body has managed to grow a baby, you can be pretty sure it also knows how to give birth!) Whenever drugs are introduced into the process, risks rise enormously and holdups are likely to occur, simply because the normal processes are disrupted.
♥ Wiithout any unnecessary drugs, you're likely to behave instinctively as you'll experience what could be called a 'cascade of hormones'. This will mean you'll know what to do when!

- ♥ When no drugs block the sensations of a baby passing through you, you're much less likely to push in the wrong way and damage yourself. Any pain is likely to be counteracted by endorphins which your body naturally produces.
- ♥ When you let your body do its thing you and your baby are both extremely alert, which is excellent for bonding. Imagine how the situation might have been if you'd met your partner while only semi-conscious or asleep...
- ♥ Your baby will also behave instinctively and will probably gaze into your eyes and then begin breastfeeding immediately. After all, he or she will probably feel a bit peckish at that point! (This is likely to continue for a few years...)
- ♥ Long-term, your baby will experience all kinds of advantages because no drugs in his or her system will have affected his or her longer-term health.
- ♥ You, yourself, will have a far, far easier time postnatally for all kinds of reasons, which of course will mean that your early days with your new baby are likely to be much more enjoyable.

If you want more detail on any of these advantages, or if you want to check out the academic research, I'm afraid you're going to have to buy another book! (*Preparing for a Healthy Birth,* ISBN: 9781906619107 provides all the information you need.) The book you're holding now is the book you need if you just want to read about a few births and feel more reassured and inspired about the whole process of pregnancy and childbirth.

Happy reading and very best wishes for an enjoyable journey into parenthood!

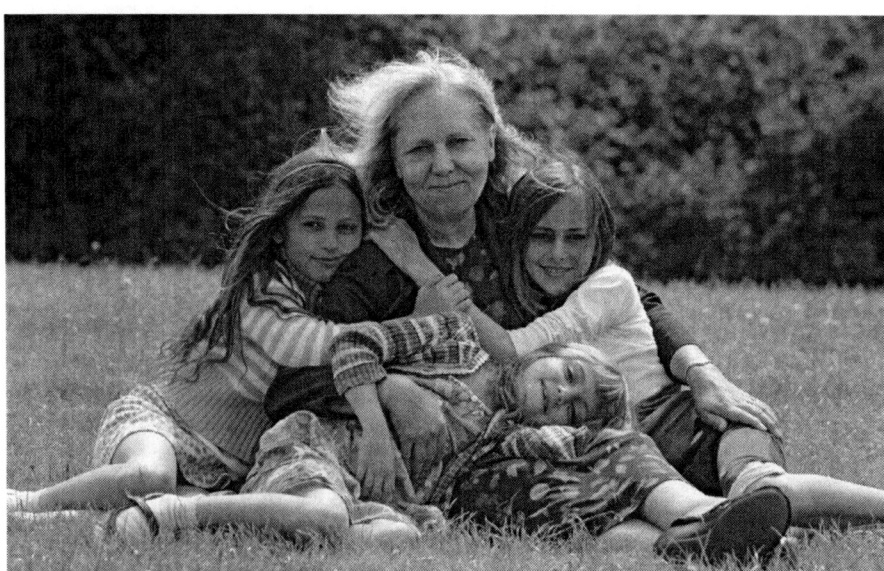

Sylvie with her three daughters, aged 7, 9 and 11

Getting pregnant...

While many babies are conceived accidentally, many others are conceived intentionally. Some couples continue working for years after meeting up and becoming committed to each other, then they suddenly realise that time is running out for them. Some couples do still have a fairytale wedding (with the white dress and the long guest list) followed by contraception-free lovemaking, in the hope that tying the knot in marriage might well lead to more. A growing minority spend years trying to conceive and eventually resort to all kinds of unnatural methods of conception, including IVF. And most of us probably do something in between, something relatively ordinary really...

When my partner and I had decided to have children we started out with a series of conversations about dates. Which would be the best date for conception, we wondered? Not only did we have to take our short-term contracts into account, we also had to consider maternity leave available to me (or not), school start dates and the benefits (or not) of our child being one of the oldest or youngest in the year. In the end, after much confusion and many disagreements about calculations we decided to just stop using contraception and see what happened. The outcome was fine, actually... I conceived in the first month of trying, miscarried a few weeks later, got pregnant again the *next* month, then eventually ended up with three girls, one who is the oldest in her year, one the youngest—and that's absolutely fine. (The maternity leave did actually work out fine for the first baby, thanks to a generous and understanding boss. The less said about the financial aspects of everything that followed, the better! Having babies is certainly not a cheap option.) Anyway, the best aspect of it all is that the three birthdays come three months apart (with my husband's birthday filling the other gap)—so we never have a problem with a glut of birthday cakes in the house!

To keep you entertained and inspired while you're trying to conceive yourself, I thought you might like to hear about a couple who took conception much more seriously than I did myself. While you enjoy the rough and tumble of undisturbed sex and grapple with any mixed emotions you might be feeling, this account might just help to remind you of the wonder and potential beauty of conception...

Candid conception

Maria Shanahan

I suppose my birth stories begin with where I was conceived, at the top of a mountain in France, St Paul de Vence. Knowing where I was conceived made me feel really special, and I was determined that when I decided to have a child, I would ask for it in the most wonderful place I could.

Other details that I was determined about were that the birth would take place in private, with only my husband present. I never had any doubt that I would have a child, or that I was totally capable of the task myself. The only person I wanted present was a beloved husband, and the concession I made to all those shocked by my plans—I was about 10 years old—was that I would allow a doctor to wait outside the door, just in case.

These convictions may have arisen out of my mother's horrific stories. She was shaved, called 'disgusting' when she inadvertently peed during labour, on her back with her legs in the air, white coats all about, and there was a categorical refusal to her request to have my father with her—he had to wait outside. All her births went uncomplicatedly, despite the hospital, and her best experience was with a home birth which she was finally allowed after my sister and I. She knew of my passion to give birth naturally and one day invited me to attend a waterbirth seminar given by Michel Odent in London. We both found him so inspiring and gentle, revolutionary really, and investigated more about waterbirths. I had always loved water and the ideas he presented seemed totally logical. A waterbirth seemed the best possible way to ease a child into the world outside the womb.

I finally met the man of my dreams when I was 27. We shared a passion for adventure and a zest for life and together determined to make our time as amazing as possible. He taught me to dive and told me of this amazing place in Oman, a place called the Tiwi Hole. It is a collapsed limestone cavern in the middle of the desert, 20 miles from the nearest village. After he had described it to me I knew it was the place—the place where we would conceive our special child: The Eye of the World.

Over to the father...

Between the mountains and the sea there is a place, a very special place. When I went there the track became tortuous as it wound steeply up off the plain, rising to a plateau riven by ancient rivers, now seldom running. The engine roared in low gear, straining to reach the top. Far away the high mountains of the Eastern Hajar rose table upon table to the clouds drawing ever closer. At last the track dropped down one last hairpinned slope to a lower plain. To the left the sea shimmered, the light of the late morning sun reflecting from rays leaping from its surface like bright diamonds of polished steel. To the right the plain rose gradually to meet the foothills preceding the majesty of the soaring heights of the Jebel. The turn-off to the right was unmarked, just the merest depressions of tyres, found only by a stirring instinct. Nothing to be seen ahead except the scrub of the plain stretching away to the hills.

Between the mountains and the sea,
there is a place, a very special place...

And then the ground opened. A huge roughly circular hole dead ahead. I brought my vehicle to a stop some way from the edge, turned the engine off and stepped out of the air-conditioned environment and into the humid silence of this land. The heat blasted stones crunched under my feet as I approached the rim and I saw a sight that would never leave me. This was the start of an adventure into more than my mind could perceive. The start to a story that ultimately would never end. I stood at the edge, my breath taken away. The ground before me long ago had collapsed into a subterranean cavern some 30m deep by 60m in diameter linked by deep channels from the sea half a mile distant to underground fresh water streams from the Jebel to the West. At the bottom, a crescent of pure turquoise water, undisturbed, reflecting in its calmness the sides of the hole.

I entered the crystal waters and dropped to a depth of 20m looking down into an impenetrable darkness to unguessed depths. Exhausted air bubbles collected in the roof of the overhang like pools of mercury. I turned away from the darkness towards the light and looked up. The rim of the hole and the water's edge formed the shape of an eye, bordered with yellow and blue. I was motionless inside this eye at the very heart of the magic, suspended in a vision looking out on the world above, through silver shafts of sunlight, which were cutting through this ether to greet me.

I broke the surface and left. I took the vision with me then and the vision held part of me there, waiting until it could show me the two people sitting at the water's edge in silence asking for their child to appear in their world.

I took the vision with me then and the vision held part of me there waiting

This place really calls to me. It is an ancient subterranean cavern, the roof of which collapsed many hundreds or even thousands of years ago. This caused a sink hole some 150 to 200 feet in diameter and about 90 feet deep. It is mainly sheer-sided and undercut on a three-quarter crescent where fresh water from beneath the mountains of the Hajar meets and mixes with salt water entering deep below via some opening to the sea which is at least quarter to a half mile away. The water is crystal clear and the most brilliant bright turquoise. In 1985, a diver recorded a depth of 55m, and he still hadn't found the bottom!

The reason I called it 'The Eye' is that at one point if you dive down to around 10 to 15m and turn back to look up to the surface, the appearance is that you are looking out through an eye which is rimmed with light blue and yellow out into another world of earth and sky. It is a unique and amazing experience once you've overcome the apprehension of being suspended within a bottomless pit!

There is such a silence of the earth here. I feel a total isolation from our everyday life of possessions and feel part of the surrounding rock, the water, the breathing wind and the silent skies. Somehow the reality of these elements runs far deeper than my normal existence as if there is some primeval relationship far beyond the reach of language. The wind from the plain above breathes around the rim with a hardly perceptible hiss dislodging the odd loose pebble which drops "plop!" into the water sending out ripples across the calm surface to the fringes of the hole. I suddenly realise what we are witnessing— the timeless erosion of the earth. At that moment my existence is thrown into a deeper perspective. Immaterial, insignificant, a newborn child in a grown-up's game. The whole span of my life might be less than the time it took the wind to excavate and dislodge the last pebble that fell into the water.

> I suddenly realise what we are witnessing—
> the timeless erosion of the earth

The Eye will always remain in our minds and the magic of the Tiwi Hole will remain with us forever between the mountains and the sea, the surface and the air.

Maria takes up the story again...

When my partner told me about this place, I visualised it so clearly... I said that this was the place where we should conceive our first child. Our dream was to ask for our child here. However, the actual practicalities of this plan were a little different from the theory!

Amassing the camping and diving equipment, as well as the four-wheel drive to get there—to be lent to us at the drop of a hat when the ovulation test strips showed positive—required a fair quantity of people to be enrolled in our plan. At last the time came and we were ready. We kitted up, wearing less than usual, and entered the water from the small shoreline. Looking past the 5 to 10m shallows, the bottom recedes into darkness under the overhanging cliff, dropping at a sharp angle to unguessed depths. I was by this time somewhat apprehensive about our planned conception. For not only was our plan to conceive here, but to actually make love at 10m whilst diving in 'The Eye'. My thoughts at this point were something along the lines of: "Oh my god, what's all that green stuff??!!", "Why are there so many little fish about??", "How far does that go down and what's lurking down there?" and "Can we seriously be considering sex down there???!!!" And although we achieved it, amazingly, the end result was not conception... probably just as well since it might have turned out to be a fish! Never had so many people been interested in my next period! Fiohann was conceived nine months later in North West London.

I was, by the time, somewhat apprehensive
about our planned conception...

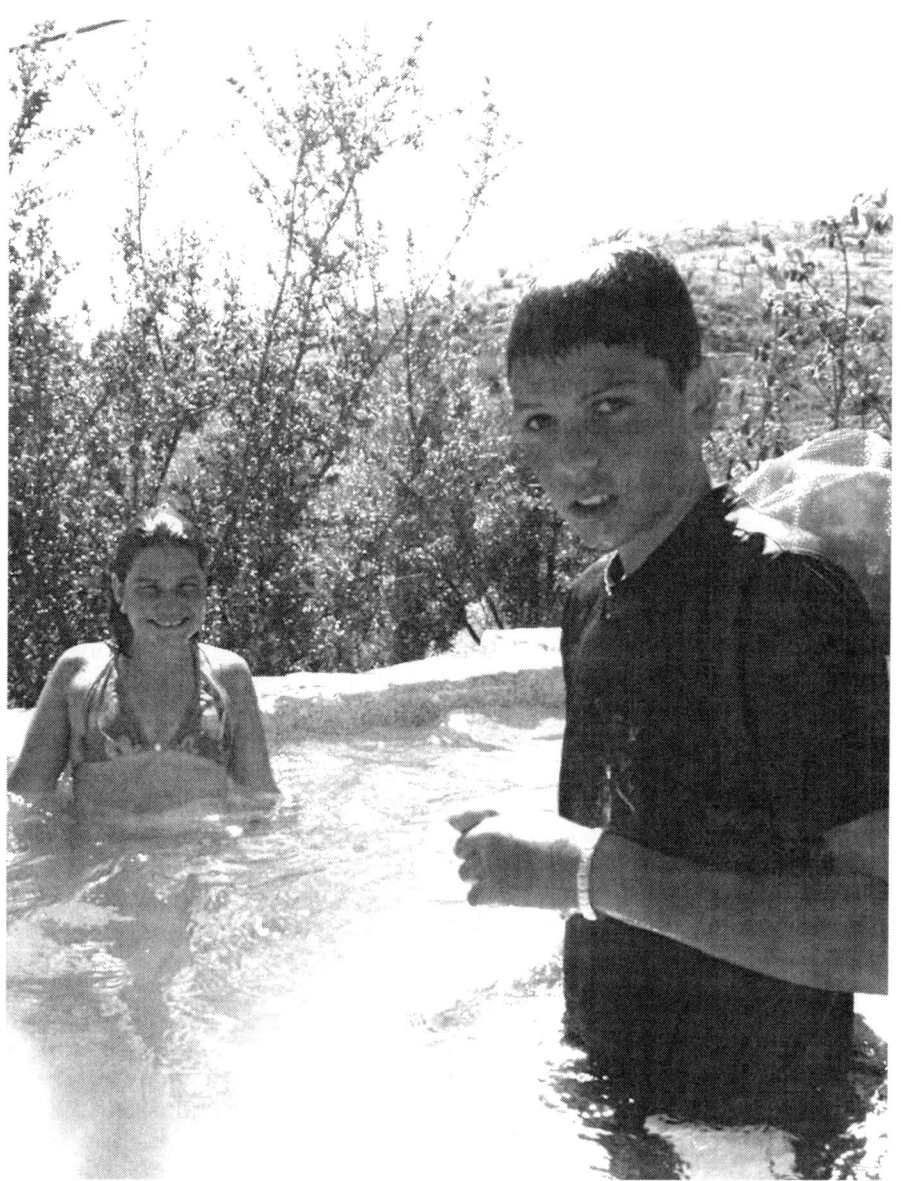

Fiohann and Eowyn, appropriately taking a dip in an open-air swimming pool!

The conception of Maria's second baby was also interesting...

My first knowledge of my daughter came when my partner and I went for dinner with friends who were desperate to find a name for their new baby girl. My friend was sure that it began with an 'E', but couldn't find the right name, so we all focused on the task at hand. By dessert we were getting close to the end of our resources... Then, from somewhere in the recesses of my mind came the name 'Eowyn'. Nevertheless, as soon as I said it, I *knew* and blurted out, "No! You can't call her that.... That's the name of my baby girl!'

Some years later, I was in a car crash and broke my arm. Quite apart from not being able to drive, Fiohann was still a toddler and needed to be carried. I went to stay with my mother so she could help me. While I was there I met an astrologer friend of hers, who wanted to have a new leaflet made so as to expand her business. I produced one for her, and she was very grateful and wanted to pay me. I refused but said instead of payment she could do my chart, even though I wasn't a great believer. When she did it I listened half heartedly, until at the end she asked if I had any questions. I asked when would be a good time to conceive our next child, since I'd been dithering. She was surprised, not normally being asked such questions. Nevertheless, she duly investigated... she said that unless I wanted to wait until I was 38—I was then 33—it would be 26 October. This was July, so I put it to the back of my mind.

26 October approached. I still dithered, thinking I was too fat, unfit, and besides, my partner and I had begun to have a rocky time. We discussed it before bed and I decided we wouldn't do it yet.

Dropping off to sleep, in that twilight zone of semi-consciousness, I suddenly heard, loud and clear, a little girl's voice saying "Now, please. Now!" I awoke suddenly and asked my partner if he'd heard it. He said he hadn't, but he had an utter conviction that now was the time. So he placed crystals that were important to him around the bed, and we made love. Very different lovemaking when you have the specific intention of creating a new life: we were more solemn and reverential about the magic of our bodies, life, creation.

We didn't make love again until we were certain, one way or the other. Sure enough, that was when she came into me and—with impeccable timing—emerged on 26 July the next year.

We didn't make love again until we were certain...

I think for me, this experience has proved to me how some things exist outside time and space and more certainly, outside our understanding. Eowyn also has a secret name, which, obviously, I can't reveal, but suffice to say it means 'spirit of the west wind'. I don't know which way the wind was blowing then, or where it will take her, but I feel incredibly privileged to be the vessel through which her spirit came to us.

Having one...

Most families only ever expect to conceive one child and even then, they usually expect the conception to be either straightforward or a surprise! When a couple eventually find themselves expecting a baby a whole new world of possibilities opens up to them and suddenly they have to climb an extremely steep learning curve as they work their way through pregnancy and all it entails. Actually, although that is a difficult journey and one well worth focusing on, we're not going to be considering it here. Instead, we're going to fast forward to the birth... and, just to make life a bit more interesting, we're going to let a man have the first word on that subject! After that, we're going to hear a woman describing the various stages of labour and we'll then hear from various other people about different birth experiences. It's all very individual, but as you'll see, there's also a bit of a pattern.

A man's view of birth

Phil Anderton

Please allow to me present my credentials: I am the father of four children, three of which were born without serious medical intervention but the last, being a breech baby, made its appearance via caesarean section. I attended all the births (three in hospital, one at home) and therefore you might think I am eminently qualified to write something on the subject of childbirth—but you'd be wrong. I am no more capable of commenting on the pros and cons of the various forms of bringing babies into the world than a professional footballer can offer advice about a good forward defensive stroke in cricket. This is simply because I am male and being male means I will never have the slightest idea of how it feels to give birth. Of course, once the line on the curious spatula thing purchased from Boots turned blue, I read books on the subject, I went to the antenatal classes more or less voluntarily and I did my best to empathise with my wife as she began to slowly swell. But no amount of lectures, films and drinks with midwives could possibly convey the actual experience of labour to those of us with a Y chromosome. This put me in a very tricky situation.

My wife has very strong views about giving birth. She wanted everything to proceed with as little medical intervention as possible and without any painkilling drugs. I could relate to this at least; personally speaking I have always had a peculiar aversion to taking pills (not even an aspirin for a hangover). Covering my face with a mask has induced panic ever since a childhood trip to a drunken dentist and allowing anyone to stick a needle into my spinal column seems like asking for trouble. But it was not me who was going to give birth, it was not me who was going to have muscles and nerves stretched to breaking point and beyond. So when she asked me for opinions on everything from arnica and other homeopathic remedies to using a TENS machine, I felt like a complete fraud offering any advice at all. To compound the problem, there was my own ignorance. I thought a TENS machine was something to do with American bowling alleys and one sip of the foul-tasting raspberry leaf tea made me feel glad I was a man. But if my sense of helpless confusion was bad during the pregnancy, things were about to get a lot worse.

I know everyone is different, but when my male friends say watching the birth of their children was one of the most rewarding experiences of their lives I can't help thinking they are either lying, complete sadists or both. How anyone can describe watching their loved ones suffer extreme pain as 'wonderful' is utterly beyond me—even when the compensation is holding your beautiful baby son or daughter in your arms. I guess the root of my problem was that there was absolutely nothing I could do during labour except to try not to get in the way. Of course, I could hold my wife's hand, offer her words of encouragement and mop her fevered brow as directed, but it all felt so inadequate.

At the time, it struck me this is why most spectators at sporting events are men. The thousands of males who flock to pitches, tracks and courses every weekend are merely in training for the day when our other halves give birth. Coping with the frustration we feel about not being able to take that crucial penalty kick, take that crucial wicket or ride that crucial winner in the 3.30 at Newmarket is excellent practice for that crucial time in the labour ward, when all we can do is stand, watch and wait. Now don't get me wrong: the midwives and medical staff were absolutely marvellous. They did their best to make me feel included and involved but nothing they said or did could alter my belief that I had contributed nothing positive to the process. I suppose this feeling of helplessness is why some men feel the need to video the births of their children—something which, in my opinion, should be punished by a life sentence of watching endless repeats of *You've Been Framed*. Playing with electronic toys is what we chaps do best and placing a lens between you and reality is an excellent way of coping with stress.

After the birth of No.1, I felt like someone who had got too drunk at a party and made a thorough nuisance of themselves, so imagine my surprise when I was invited back, again, and again, and again! Did it get easier? Yes and no. Every birth is different but the risks remain the same. There is the worry that you are pushing your luck and that something may go horribly wrong. However, the other side of the coin is that the relief gets greater every time it goes right.

So did I do anything right? I suppose I must have done because I am still married to the mother of my four healthy children and she never, not even during our bitterest rows, refers to any mistakes I made during her confinements. If I did contribute anything positive it was, paradoxically, not what I did but what I didn't do. I did not insist she have a natural childbirth but once she had made her decision to do so, I did not insist she stick to it—note the medically necessary caesarean required to deliver No.4. I did not allow my natural inclination to 'take charge' get the better of me. Instead, I let my wife and the midwives take the decisions and get on with it. The 'did not' I am most proud of, though, is that I did not squeal like a stuck pig when she dug her nails into my arm!

I was happy enough to do exactly as I was told but equally my wife knew she had my support whatever her decision. For example, No.2 was three weeks late and the doctors were keen to induce the birth artificially. However, the baby was showing no signs of distress and my wife wanted to wait. If it had been me I would have wanted to be hooked up to every available machine in the hospital... but it wasn't me. I therefore shut up so my wife could listen to what her body was telling her. Our (or should I say her) reward was a bouncing, baby boy weighing an eye-watering 10lb 2oz (!) and delivered without any drugs or intervention.

Why, you may ask, if I found the births so distressing did I allow myself to be persuaded to attend? Some of you reading this may like to pick up on my earlier football analogy and ask why men spend hours in the wet and cold cheering on a bunch of overpaid, prima donnas, but I would prefer to sum up the whole experience in a single word. I bit the metaphorical bullet, swallowed my pride and allowed myself to be 'persuaded' into taking decisions against my male judgement for one reason and one reason only: it's called 'love'.

The stages of labour

Angela Horn

Onset of labour...

My second baby was due on 5 or 6 June. I was enjoying late pregnancy and was taken by surprise when he decided to arrive a week and a half early

Friday, 26 May, lunchtime: had a show. Didn't notice this last time, but no mistaking this one—a large blob of jelly. Realise this means baby could arrive any time between this day and two weeks, and hope it's nearer two weeks as baby isn't due until 6 June. I want him to 'cook' as long as he needs, and I *like* late pregnancy—and I have things to do!

Drive to my good friend Wendy's home in South West London (1 hour 15 minute journey each way) so my son, Lee, can exhaust her toddler instead of exhausting me. Maybe not a good idea in retrospect, but I wanted to carry on as if nothing was happening. Memo to self: next time you have *any* signs of approaching labour, get some rest!! I have period-type pains on way home—hoping nothing will happen for a few days though. Lee decides to be extremely hyperactive all evening and is quite a handful. My husband, Graham, says Lee is like the actor Brian Blessed, i.e. his preferred volume in any conversation is a loud SHOUT. I feel cold in the evening, but do not realise its significance—my mother has told me that animals usually have a temperature drop as labour approaches. At midnight I am knackered and am still having period-type pains. I rub rose oil on my tummy—I know some people think it brings on contractions, but I feel a strong 'craving' for it. Lee is still going strong. At 12.30 I'm breastfeeding him to try to get him to settle down to sleep, thinking "I really hope I don't go into labour tonight", when there's a big gush of fluid. It smells salty and sweet—definitely amniotic fluid—and, fortunately, is clear.

First stage...

I tell Graham that the baby is likely to be born within the next 24 hours, and—I think shortly afterwards—I notice mild contractions every four minutes. Graham (after a few glasses of wine earlier in the evening) gets extremely excited and starts putting up the birth pool. He suggests he read me Harry Potter stories through the labour to distract me. A lovely idea, but I don't fancy it at the moment! Lee *eventually* goes to sleep and I check progress with the pool. Graham has assembled it upside-down. He starts again. Contractions still very mild, really like Braxton-Hicks, so I'm hoping the baby might wait until tomorrow. Before long the pool is assembled, I've made sure that everything I need is in the sitting room with the pool, turned on immersion heater, checked the animals all have food and water, and can focus on the task in hand.

Contractions still mild but regular. I phone the labour ward at Greenwich to say that I'm booked for a homebirth with Vicky of Garland team, and am in early labour. "Oh no…" says the lady on the phone. Apparently they are snowed under and Vicky is on duty in the ward for the third night in a row, but she will get her to call me. Vicky calls back and says she'll come out to assess me whenever I want. She stresses that homebirth bookings take priority so she will leave the labour ward whenever it's necessary.

I don't know when I want her to come out—it all seems very mild, but I have no idea how fast a second labour might progress. My first was nine hours and very steady. I decide to try to get some sleep and say I'll call Vicky again if things seem to step up a gear.

We go to bed at 2.30am—Graham falls fast asleep (lucky git), while I lie on my side with hot water bottles, having contractions every four minutes and finding them increasingly uncomfortable. Doze in between. Give up at 3.30am as need to be on all fours for contractions. Look at Lee sleeping (we have a huge family bed) and feel a little sad that it will no longer be just me and him.

I ask Vicky to examine me. She says there's no need, but she will if I want. I want her to because I think I'll be really far along, but I'm only 3cm dilated. This is a surprise as, when I was in labour with Lee, I'm sure the contractions weren't this much work at the one time I was examined, and I was 4-5cm then.

Vicky reminds me that with second labours, a vaginal examination doesn't tell you much as you can ping open very quickly—and I think this is why she didn't really want to do one. During the examination, Vicky noted that the bag of waters was still bulging in front of the baby's head, so the large gush of fluid I had earlier was a hindwater leak. I am glad to hear this as it means that the forewaters could still provide valuable cushioning for the baby's head during the labour.

I stay in the sitting room with just a lava lamp for dim lighting, and music on quietly. I use a birth ball (large inflatable rubber ball, about 18" diameter) for a couple of contractions, leaning over it and rocking round and round. But mainly I have to be on all fours, rocking, circling my hips, and humming. I focus on breathing out slowly and calmly during contractions and just let breathing happen of its own accord.

Contractions still don't seem to last an awfully long time, nor do they seem to be changing much—still hard work, but at no point in this labour are they ever as hard as the worst ones in my first labour, nor as mild as the milder ones at the start of it. The sensation is quite different, too—until transition/second stage last time I felt contractions more as intense muscular effort than what I would call 'pain', but these feel more like pain under my bump. I try to relax and breathe through the tension, but feel that lack of sleep is responsible for a lot of the discomfort—and perhaps my attitude, since I really do feel cheated of a night's sleep! Why couldn't it have waited until morning??!

I am aware in the labour that my attitude will affect the way I feel contractions, so I do try to focus on every contraction bringing my baby closer, and my body opening like a flower, etc, etc... A song I was listening to yesterday is stuck in my head—Jefferson Airplane, or are they called Starship by this time? Don't know the title but there is a line about "There are children being born who will amaze you...". Blame my parents for this—I was brought up in the hippy tradition! Anyway, I love that song in labour... in my head (and sometimes in my body) I am singing it and thinking of those children being born! I also think of an image which helps me to focus on my breathing, which I have always practised when doing yoga. As I breathe in, I visualise the branches of a tree growing rapidly, as in time-lapse photography, and I think about freeing my neck and spine upwards and forwards. As I breathe out, I visualise the roots of the tree spreading through the ground, growing as I watch, and think about relaxing downwards, if that makes sense. I don't want to sound like a complete airhead or dippy hippy here, because really I'm not—honest!—but this really does help with contractions. As with last time, I really value the gaps between contractions when I feel clear-headed and just 'me'. Entonox ('gas and air') is available in the midwife's birth kit, but I don't want to use it as I won't risk anything affecting my state of mind. I just want to deal with contractions as they happen and to enjoy the rests in between.

I won't risk anything affecting my state of mind

At about 8am the contractions start to feel different—not 'pushy' yet, but a lot harder, and I feel joint pain in my pelvis—my sacro-iliac joints, I think. I know this means big progress and that the baby is really moving down. Soon I start to feel 'pre-pushy', i.e. no urge to push yet but I can tell it won't be long. Vicky asks if I feel any urge to push; no, and I explain that I'm determined not to do any deliberate pushing, just to let my body decide on its own and to only push when I can't stop myself. Contractions are becoming very hard work and I'm having to hum ("Ommmmm...") and moan through them. Antonia, Lee's godmother, arrives between contractions and I immediately ask her to check Lee as I think I heard him waking.

Second stage...

At some time towards 8.30 I start getting irresistible pushing urges so I go with the flow, only pushing when my body does it involuntarily, and keeping quiet in between. At this point, Vicky starts asking "Are you feeling any urge to push?" I don't manage to reply but am thinking "What do you THINK I'm doing?" The backup midwife, Rose, arrives at 8.30. Vicky is asking me to come over to be examined, and do I want to sit on a stool, and do I feel any urge yet, and can we bail some water out as it's too deep to deliver in if I'm staying on all fours... I hear her asking Rose and what about long gloves, and I am wondering what on earth she wants gloves for, since she won't be needing to have her hands in the water! I studiously ignore all this, as I am getting on with the job of giving birth and know *exactly* what I am doing! I do manage to say "No" when Vicky asks if she can examine me. Wonders of a birth pool: no one can get near you to examine you without your cooperation! I just edge backwards towards Graham with each contraction so he can rub my back. (Graham says later that it was completely obvious to him that the baby was going to be born soon regardless, so he didn't know why Vicky was bothering!)

I pull myself upright with hands on the edge of the birth pool, kneeling upright on the floor—just like last time. Feel baby's head moving down. Feel the head crowning. The head feels like it's one third of the way out, but I'm not deliberately pushing. The contraction ends and I feel that 'ring of fire' continuing—it's so hard not to push when I know that one good shove would get the head out and stop the burning, but I don't. Another contraction, another lull, more relaxing and panting, then another, and the head is born. More burning, another wait for the body. Vicky is worrying about the baby's head hitting the floor of the pool. I'm thinking "Stop fussing, woman. I know what I'm doing". I semi-stand up to deliver the body and see hands reaching for my baby. I say "Don't grab the baby!" and keep hold of him. I stand up fully, and out comes a baby! I don't think that the midwife is trying to take the baby, by the way. She is just there in case he needs to be 'caught'. I should have explained in my birth plan how I would like the second stage to be managed— ideally with the midwife just sitting and watching. I don't realise until this birth quite how I would feel about this sort of thing.

I semi-stand up to deliver the body...
I stand up fully, and out comes a baby!

I stand up and cuddle the baby, immediately check the sex and see that it's a boy. I tell Graham. I remember noticing a little mucus in his nose and mouth, so I hold him leaning forward over my arm so that it can drain—which it does, quickly and easily. I think of sitting down in the pool again for a rest, but decide to get out and have a nice comfy chair. Antonia brings Lee downstairs—he has just woken up and he sees his brother just seconds after the birth. I look down at the pool and see that the water is clear—hey, no blood! Does that mean no tears?

I get out of the pool, sit down on the sofa and cuddle my baby, with Lee on the other side—feeling thrilled, very 'buzzy'—that post-birth euphoria. (I didn't get that at all last time—I felt 'high' during the labour, but a little flat after the birth. Not this time.) Am thrilled with my baby, but he looks so small. I am determined not to be separated from him. We sit down and Vicky comes over to check on us.

My other friend, Wendy, arrives—with her husband Haydon and toddler Monica, as well as her baby, which I wasn't expecting. With several good friends here, it is as if we have a post-birth party! However, the house does seem quite crowded with two midwives and all our visitors. In future I will be careful to preserve the intimacy of the family at this special time immediately after the birth. It is very nice for me, sitting there cuddling my lovely newborn, but I feel now that Graham, Lee, Robert and I would have benefited from a little private time together as a family, before the birth is celebrated with our friends.

Third stage...

I have planned a physiological (drug-free) third stage on the understanding that the midwife will administer drugs [syntometrine] if she is worried about my bleeding. I ask Vicky not to clamp the cord as I want to wait until the placenta is delivered, which she is perfectly happy with. (One big advantage of this is that your baby has to stay cuddled up to you the whole time—enforced bonding! No one can take him away to be weighed and measured and fussed over, leaving you to get on with the messy and boring part...)

I am not looking forward to the third stage as last time it took over an hour, but this time I am much more aware of contractions and push properly with them. I try squatting and feel like I want to go to the loo. Oh no, I manage to avoid crapping in the birth pool but now I am going to do it on the floor! Vicky says that will just be the placenta and to push, but I don't believe her. It's only about 10 minutes after the birth, and surely it can't all be over that quickly? However, a little push and there it is—with just a tiny smidgen of blood (estimated 100ml). Is that it? Amazingly easy!

Cutting the cord...

The cord is tied with string, not a hard plastic clamp, and Graham cuts it.

The cord is tied with string, not a hard plastic clamp

Immediately after the birth...

I keep the baby with me while Vicky checks him, then I grudgingly let go of him for a minute as he is weighed. Only 8lb—a lot smaller than Lee's 9lb 6oz, although with 11 more days to go he would probably have been bigger, had he held on.

Procedures for the mother...

One thing I was sure of—I was keen to avoid tearing and, in the event, I knew what to do on my own. Vicky examines me and—hooray!—no tears or even grazes. Women, this intact perineum thing is great! Wendy and Haydon crack open some champagne they've brought with them and Vicky offers to get us some breakfast. I think she should be getting some sleep instead!

Breastfeeding and beyond...

Five weeks later: Robert is a wonderful baby, very calm and contented. I'm aware that this may change later!

He is a very efficient feeder, is growing well, and sleeps well at night. Because we have a family bed, there have been no sleepless nights so far— I just feed him on my side lying down, frequently falling asleep while doing so, and he wakes maybe once or twice a night for a guzzle. Long may it continue! During the day he follows a fairly normal newborn breastfeeding pattern, which involves feeding perhaps every hour or so, and occasionally goes for two hours while sleeping. This may sound like a lot, but it's perfectly normal because the newborn's stomach is so small and breastmilk so easily digested. It's no trouble at all as I usually feed him in an over-the-shoulder sling and can do it while reading a book or walking around.

I'm still breastfeeding Lee (my toddler) briefly, a couple of times a day, and I've fed him and Robert together a few times—quite hard to arrange, but cute. Lee is amazingly gentle with Robert so far, and likes to stroke his head while they feed together, or to cuddle Robert while he is feeding. I hope it carries on this way and am very glad I'm still feeding Lee as it seems a great way to reassure him that I still love him and to spend close time with him. I am counting my blessings and feeling very lucky.

Robert is a wonderful baby, very calm and contented. I'm aware that this may change later!

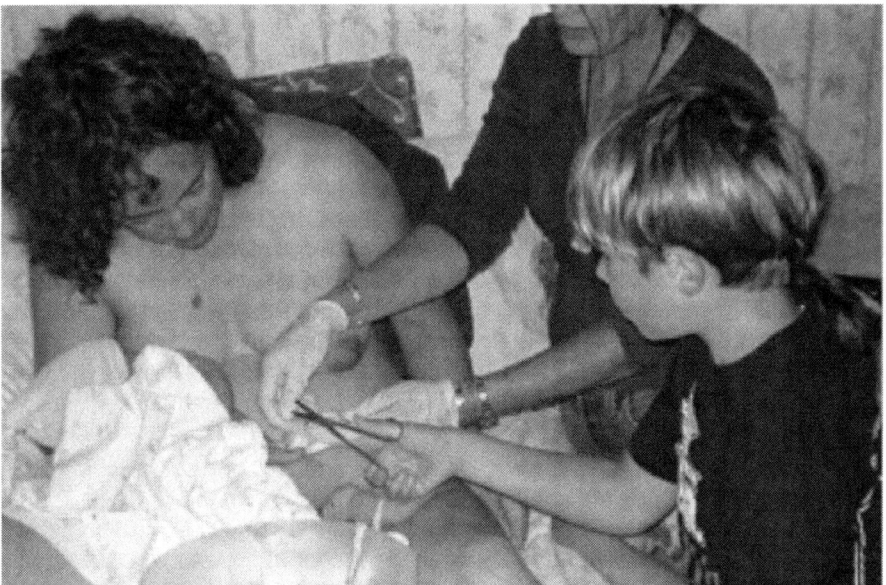

Cutting the cord

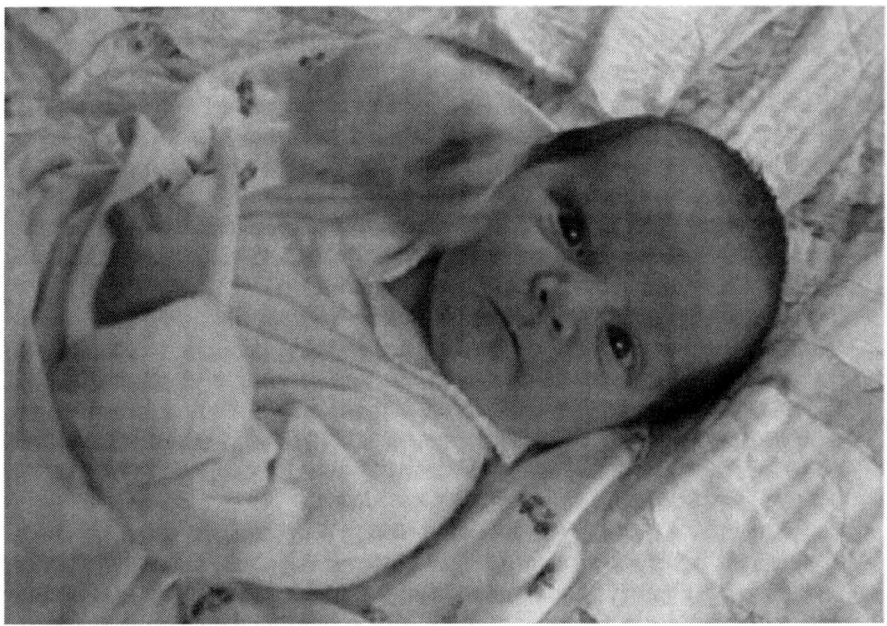

An alert newborn baby after a physiological birth. Babies who are born without any drugs in their system are extremely alert and keen to take in all that they find around them—especially people, and in particular their new mum and dad!

Does birth have to be painful?

Sylvie Donna

As I said before, birth isn't necessarily painful for women, but it usually is. I suppose it's not really surprising because a very large 'object' (oh, all right then, a *baby*) needs to travel through a passageway which just isn't used to accommodating anything of that size. Nevertheless, it's well worth remembering that hormones have an enormous influence on our bodies. And we're used to sexual processes having an effect on size, aren't we? Just as a man's penis becomes bigger under certain circumstances (which is what got us onto this whole subject in the first place), a woman's vagina becomes bigger during the process of birth... and just like a man's penis, it shrinks back to normal size afterwards! Even with this logic, I can understand it if you're worried about the prospect of this process going well and about the pain factor.

Actually, when it comes to birth, there are some very good reasons for the sensations, even if they are painful and *extremely* painful in many cases. There are also good reasons not to be too fearful and it's reassuring to know that your mind and body adapts naturally when you labour in an undrugged state...

♥ When you labour undrugged and *undisturbed*, (under the discrete care of a well-qualified midwife, for example), you are likely to drift off into another state of mind—just as you might do when you're having sex—and your body will produce endorphins to counteract the pain. This is why so many women who have a healthy labour and birth report a real postnatal high.

♥ Any 'extreme' sensations make labour smoother, easier and *less* painful because moving to a more comfortable position (which is what you're likely to do) also helps the baby to get into an appropriate position and descend, as necessary, for the birth. Bearing in mind that there is actually no such thing as a painless birth (since epidurals can't cover the whole of labour and caesareans involve postnatal pain) a smoother, easier and therefore *shorter* labour has got to be good news, hasn't it?

♥ If you experience the sensations of labour without any drug-based pain relief, I am convinced you will actually experience less pain overall. This is quite simply because all drugs have side-effects and after-effects. Therefore, women who've used drugs almost always have a much worse time postnatally (both physically and emotionally) than women who've had entirely healthy births. Nowadays, people seem to expect things to be difficult after the birth... but they really needn't be.

♥ Experiencing an unmanaged labour—which is only possible when no drugs are involved—is much more dignified for you so will cause you no *emotional* pain. Compare being bedridden with legs akimbo, to being up and about, and giving birth in any position at all, with a minimum of people around—preferably just one midwife. Emotionally, it's a million times less traumatic.

In any case, some women really do experience labour and birth as positive...

I wouldn't call the sensations 'pain'

Angela Horn

The pain of the contractions themselves was more just a sensation of intense muscular effort—uncomfortable, but not sharp pain, like any other form of exertion in sport or physical work. I wouldn't call the sensations of *contractions* 'pain', although they did need to be dealt with. However, that is not meant to imply that I had no pain in labour! For me, the hardest part was early second stage. The pain I had was joint pain—sharp, shooting pains in my hips, as though the joints were being stretched. Graham said later that he could see my hips moving apart, almost bulging out of their sockets. Although the peaks of these contractions hurt a lot, during the pauses between contractions I felt fine but tired, and the intensity of each contraction built up gradually so that I had plenty of time to get myself onto all fours, call Graham to start rubbing my back and to turn the music up. This predictability made the pain easier to manage. I also knew that each contraction would only go on for a finite time—even during really intense periods when the contractions were close together, there would be a break between them, however short. It also helped to remember that this pain was positive pain—that strong contractions meant things were moving along. This pain was telling me how not to hinder my body—no surprise that labour is harder to bear in the positions which make it harder for the baby to be born, such as lying on your back. At no stage did I ask for pain relief, or want it—although at one point I remember thinking "OK, I've done natural childbirth now. Next time maybe I'll try a caesarean"! The midwife later commented that I must have a high pain threshold. Balls! It still hurt, I just dealt with it in my own way. It hurts, but pain itself doesn't kill you and you soon get over it. I was far more afraid of losing control than of pain—of losing control of my mind through fear, panic or mind-altering drugs, and of losing control of the situation through medical intervention.

On the day, I had a wonderful midwife, I was in my own home with my husband and I had nothing to worry about. I had gone to great lengths to make sure that I was fit and healthy, and to the best of our knowledge the baby was healthy too. In the face of all these positive factors, pain seems such a transient thing—like homesickness or feeling lovesick. You can reassure yourself that it *will* get better and that soon you will feel normal again. It was easy for me to be calm. I did not feel afraid at any point. I was on my own territory—if there was anything I did not like about my environment, I could change it (or ask someone else to) without asking anyone's permission. No one could tell me what to do, and no one was going to start treating me like a child. For me personally, I'm sure it would have been much harder in a hospital room, where all I could focus on was the labour and whether the hospital's procedures or policies were going to affect it.

The pain itself doesn't kill you, and you soon get over it

My longest labours were four hours

Debbie Shaw

I have always had a lot of contact with babies and children. I have a half sister and brother who are 12 and 18 years younger than I am. I met my children's father when I was 18 and he had a young daughter who we often had to stay with us. I enjoyed looking after children when I was younger and always wanted to have a baby myself. I now have five children: Hannah, Faye, Liam, Ashley and Luke.

All my births have been relatively easy. My longest labours were four hours with my first and fourth children. The shortest labour was one hour with my third child. There were no major complications during any of my labours, although I did have to have stitches after each birth. I also bled quite heavily afterwards. My second child became distressed during labour because the cord was wrapped twice around her neck, restricting her breathing. She was given oxygen immediately after delivery. I never used any pain relief during any of my labours, there was never time anyway. I was encouraged to try gas and air during my first labour, but this made me vomit.

I assume my labours were quick and easy compared to other women due to genes. My mother also had quick, easy labours. [Comment from Sylvie: Other women have told me their mothers had long, difficult labours. Could there be another reason for women having fast labours?] I never did anything special in any of my pregnancies to help myself give birth easily. I did have a positive attitude towards labour and was not worried at the prospect of giving birth.

I had all my babies in hospital.
The baby's father also preferred that.

I had all my babies in hospital. I did want a home birth with my fourth child, but was told that because I was anaemic it was not advisable in case I bled heavily. The baby's father also preferred the baby to be born in hospital. This labour began with a show, followed almost immediately by mild contractions. These became stronger and close together quite quickly. I stayed at home for the first two hours and, when I felt I needed the support of a midwife, was taken to the hospital. The midwife consulted with me throughout labour and allowed me to make the decisions for my care. My waters broke after about an hour and the baby was delivered normally about an hour later, after just three pushes.

With my fifth child, the midwife actually suggested a possible home birth the first time I met her. However, she said I would have to change my doctor temporarily as the practice I was registered with did not support home births. I decided to have the baby in hospital but was provided with a home birth pack and advice in case I didn't make it to the hospital.

This labour started with quite strong contractions almost immediately. They became very frequent after about an hour. I had to wait for someone to arrive to look after my other children. I arrived at the hospital 10 minutes before I delivered the baby. Shortly after my arrival at the hospital my waters broke and the baby arrived almost immediately after one push. I was allowed home six hours later.

I don't regret having my babies in hospital, although I would like to have experienced a home birth. Since I had my first child, care for pregnant women has improved. The woman has more choice with regard to labour and I found there was much less medical interference.

Even though the choices are there I still think there is room for improvement to encourage women to make these choices. Until my last pregnancy I was never offered a choice of where to have my babies. I had to ask. Even with my last pregnancy when I was offered a choice there was still the problem of the GP practice I was with not being willing to support this choice.

Of course I still go to the gym!

Anon

Once I found out I was pregnant I wanted to make sure that I did everything possible to help me with the labour. I was 36 but it was becoming the trend to have babies later in life so I didn't really think about my age. Whilst trying for a baby I took folic acid, as recommended. I did have quite bad sickness for the first three months or so but once that was over I kept as fit as possible. I had always regularly attended a gym and generally used to keep fit and active so couldn't see any reason to change that. I used to enjoy weight training but obviously changed to much lighter weights and started swimming a lot more. A friend of mine had swum regularly throughout her pregnancy and had quite an easy labour so I decided to follow her example. I went to the gym three times a week throughout my pregnancy and swam twice a week. I swam up to 40 lengths at a time, obviously getting slower as my pregnancy advanced! This was the breaststroke, incidentally, which Sylvie tells me would have helped the baby get into a good position for the birth.

I ate as healthily as possible and bought a blender to make fruit smoothies to up my intake of fruit. Constipation is sometimes an unwelcome side effect of pregnancy! I also read an article in a magazine about raspberry leaf tea, which is a herbal remedy and is supposed to help shorten labour. I had nothing to lose so decided to try this too, taking it in tablet form, which I preferred. Each tablet was 400mg and the label said to have one 3 to 6 times a day. It said the tablet could also be broken up and dissolved in hot water—but it tasted awful this way! It seems raspberry leaf is recommended for the last three months of pregnancy but not before. I also read that rubbing Vitamin E oil onto your perineum regularly can help stretch this area and lessen the chance of having to be cut whilst giving birth. Again, I thought "Why not?" so I used to massage the oil in every night throughout the last six to eight weeks.

I worked full-time right up to seven days before giving birth and although I was tired toward the end I am glad I did because I believe it is important to keep active for as long as possible. The baby arrived three days before my due date. At 10 o'clock at night my waters broke naturally. I was at home and I had no warning at all—I just got up from my chair to take a glass into the kitchen and that was it! I was relatively calm and was in no pain or discomfort whatsoever. I gathered my bags and got to the hospital for around 11 o'clock. At about 1.00am I started getting contractions—they were quite strong and started coming regularly. It seemed to happen very quickly and I was a bit shocked at how strong they were. At about 3.00am the nurses on the delivery ward examined me and discovered I was around 7cm dilated. I was quite shocked and things started happening very, very quickly by then. The contractions just got stronger and stronger and by about 3.45am I was fully dilated. I had decided beforehand that I wanted to try and squat to give birth and not lie flat on my back but I found that I was not really strong enough because it is very hard on the thighs! The nurses raised the bed up so that I was practically sitting and I had both feet on the bed, which was a huge help. I gave birth at 4.10am, exactly 1 hour 10 minutes after arriving in the delivery suite. I was totally alert and felt absolutely wonderful, apart from being a bit sore. I had no stitches at all, just a graze, which healed itself. The whole experience was amazing.

My body healed very quickly indeed and I had no problems whatsoever. I was back at the gym 10 days later and regained my figure very quickly. I am sure that my easy labour was a direct result of the preparation I did throughout my pregnancy.

How am I going to say no?

Jenny Sanderson

When I was pregnant with my first child, and in a state of almost total ignorance about childbirth, my husband Tim and I attended Active Birth antenatal classes. I retained very little of the information we were given but will never forget the assertiveness role-play we did. It seemed that a hospital birth would involve countless interventions that had to be resisted—and I knew that I would not be able to resist them.

Then a friend told me about a lecture by Michel Odent that she had attended and suggested I phone him; he lived in London and delivered babies at home. So as not to disappoint her, rather than anything else, I called and made an appointment.

It was all very straightforward—my pregnancy was normal, he was available around the time I was due and, almost before I realised it, we had arranged for him to deliver me at home.

My Active Birth teacher, surprisingly, was concerned. How would I cope just with my husband, Tim, as a labour companion? Did I know that Michel would pretty well leave us to it? This didn't seem like a problem to me compared with the treatment I seemed certain to get and the battles we'd have to fight in hospital. And it was the right choice for me. Rebecca was born after a straightforward if not an easy labour. Rosamund was born the following year, also at home with Michel. Two (and a few years later that would be four) healthy births. No continuous monitoring, no vaginal examinations, no episiotomies, no tears, no syntometrine, no hospital food...

Michel's calm confidence in the labour process and in the labouring woman encouraged me, and his extensive experience reassured me that everything was normal. I knew that he would know at once if there was a problem. If he wasn't in the room with me, he was within earshot and very much aware of what was happening—although he left me mostly to find my own way.

The labour itself

On the morning of my EDD [expected date of delivery] I didn't feel too good, not very well but not bad enough to cancel friends who were coming to lunch—an arrangement deliberately made for this date, on the assumption that the first baby would be 'late'. I ate a normal breakfast.

Our friends arrived about 11.00am. Soon after, I began to feel that I didn't want to sit still and went round the garden and up and down the house. We called Michel; I spoke to him but he wasn't anxious, especially when he heard about the breakfast. By lunchtime, I didn't want to be sociable or to eat anything and went upstairs. Tim phoned Michel again and everyone had lunch, leaving by early afternoon just as Michel arrived. He saw that I was not in 'hard labour', felt the baby's heartbeat and pronounced everything to be normal.

During the afternoon and early evening I spent some of my time walking round the bedroom but mostly in the bath or on the toilet. Later on I found leaning against the towel rail useful but I didn't want to use Tim for support and the one time I tried lying down on some cushions felt stranded and found the contractions harder to manage. I spent a good deal of time on the toilet, though I'm sure my bowels were long since empty.

I found leaning against the towel rail useful

During this time Michel listened to the baby's heartbeat several times with his Doppler machine and confirmed that the mucous plug had been ejected into the bath. He spent most of the time upstairs in the spare room with a book and occasionally talking to Tim.

Shortly after 8.00pm Michel could hear that my breathing had turned to grunting and suggested that I move out of the bathroom into the bedroom. Tim supported me for two or three contractions before Rebecca was born at 8.25pm, by candlelight. Michel laid her on a towel and used his mucus extractor. Then Rebecca and I lay down on some cushions. She didn't want to breastfeed but didn't cry much either. Michel lay on our bed for half an hour or so; Tim made drinks. At about 9.00pm I delivered the placenta into a hastily found casserole dish; we did not eat it! Michel weighed Rebecca (8lb) and did the necessary paperwork before leaving us to a leisurely meal.

> I delivered the placenta into
> a hastily found casserole dish. We did not eat it!

The next morning he returned and we phoned the hospital, my doctor and the midwives. Michel and a midwife visited for most of the following 10 days.

My second labour

About three days after my second baby was due I went out in the afternoon with Rebecca (my first daughter), experiencing occasional indigestion-like twinges. By the time Tim came home I thought I was probably in labour but didn't mention it until about 6.30 or 7.00pm. We put Bec to bed and I phoned Michel at around 8.30pm; this time he said he'd come straight away. Tim and I then had dinner, though I ate only moderately. After Michel arrived we had a cup of tea. Tim and I went for a short walk and when I returned I went at once to the bath, where I stayed for most of the rest of the labour.

From about 10.15pm contractions were getting very strong. At approx. 10.40pm I thought I needed to go to the loo, but after straining for a bit, I reached down and felt the head. Rosamund was born all in one go with the next contraction, at 10.45pm; Michel caught her as she came out and laid her on a towel.

I lay in the bathroom with the baby for half an hour or so and then squatted to deliver the placenta with no assistance. Michel checked me, weighed Ros (7½lb) and did his paperwork before leaving us together.

This labour was certainly the shortest. I was out visiting friends at about 5.00pm when I felt the first early contractions and Ros was born just over five hours later. There obviously was a second stage but it was very short and I didn't need to do any strenuous pushing as I did for the other three. But it was quite a shock for the baby to be born so quickly.

> I was out visiting friends at about 5.00pm when I felt
> the first contractions and Ros was born just over five
> hours later. The second stage was very short.

My third and fourth labours

For me there were overwhelming advantages in having home births and I went on to have two more (which, unfortunately, Michel was unable to attend) with an excellent midwife. [These were two more normal, healthy births.]

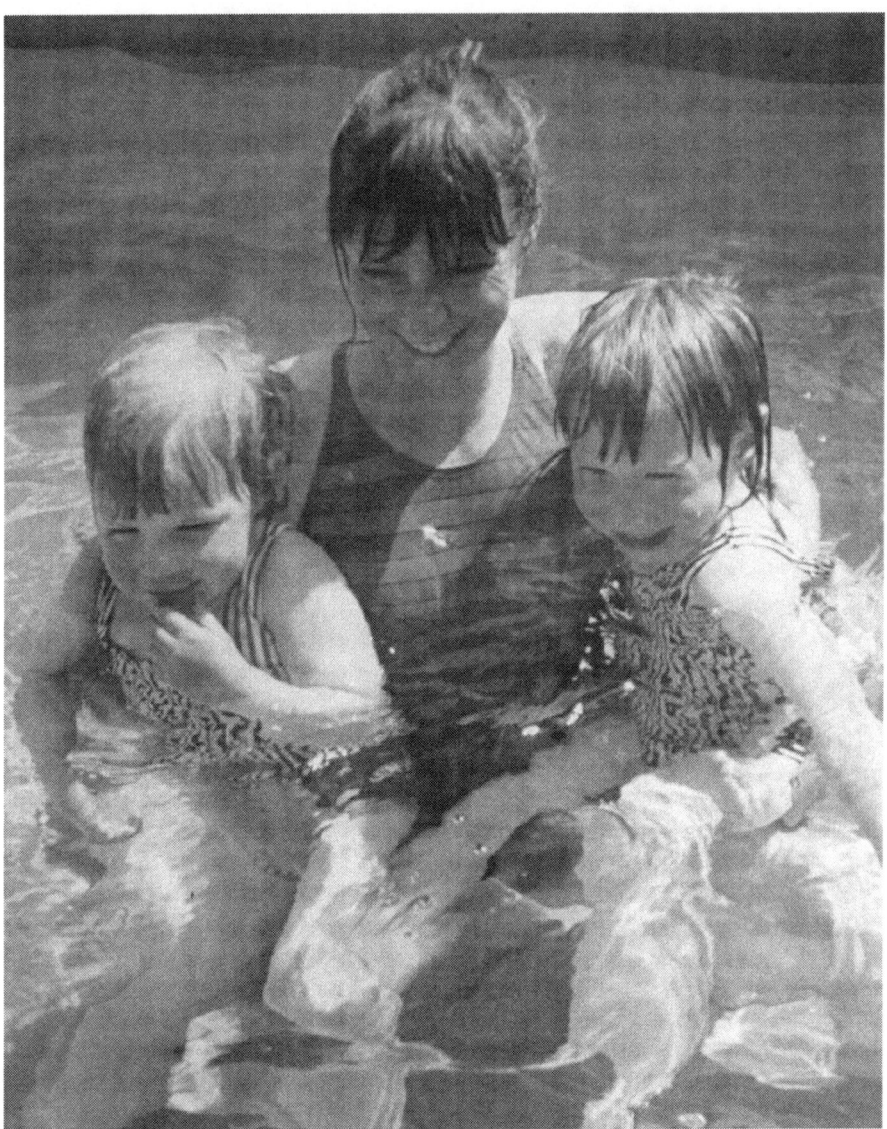

Jenny with two of her children

Having a doula

Natalie Meddings

It was an 11th-hour decision to have a doula at the birth of my second child. For eight months, my plan was to go to a local birth centre, as I had for my first. And then as if by magic, a new trust arrived in me. One that told me I could manage at home. It really was a kind of magic. My head didn't convince me, or even my heart. Just as with my first pregnancy, an imaginary hand appeared— deep-down instinct, I suppose—and I took hold of it.

As it turned out, that hand wasn't so imaginary. Two months before my due date, I attended a doula course with Liliana Lammers and Michel Odent. I found their ideas on birth exciting—at times breathtakingly so. I was especially fascinated by their belief in total privacy as being the key to a smooth birth and when Liliana helped me set up a home birth for myself, I knew she was the one I wanted by my side. As it turned out, she offered me more than that. This wonderfully calm and centred doula was more about and behind me, than beside me. Unseen, silent—but absolutely there.

I was over two weeks late and pressure was mounting to get things going. Forget induction. Liliana had convinced me that even gentler nudges, like a sweep or reflexology were to miss the point. It must be the baby that gives the cue, she explained. "If the baby is ready, then the birth will go well." She urged me to feel for myself if everything was OK. Assured me that as the mother, I would know if something was wrong. I'd hang up the phone and feel a fresh energy. Something sure and strong and safe, guiding me. What Liliana was leading me to was my own instinct.

[Note here that doulas are generally advised not to provide *advice* to pregnant women. Doulas need to tread a fine line between helping women and standing aside.]

Finally, at 5.00am on a dark November morning, I felt the first twinge. By 9.00am, labour was really established and my husband, Danny, called Liliana. In true style, there was no urgency, no panic. She said she'd see to a couple of things, then cycle over mid-morning. Her ease was contagious. I did some cleaning, made some breakfast—calmly absorbing that most unabsorbable of notions. That at some point that day, I'd have my baby in my arms.

As soon as Liliana arrived, around midday, she made herself scarce— practising absolutely what she and Michel preached. I remember wanting to offer her tea, to make her comfortable, to talk—but she just shushed me and I closed my eyes. As I moved from room to room, from kneeling to standing and back again, I looked like someone alone. But Liliana was there all right. I could feel her unmistakable energy beaming through the walls. Could feel her listening—keeping an eye.

I could feel Liliana's unmistakable energy

What I wasn't was being watched. I was totally private—and right inside myself as a result. Danny had made himself scarce, the house was silent, the room I'd somehow guided myself to, small and dark, and the world just fell away. I felt absolutely safe, wholly secure in my surroundings and the chemicals just cued themselves up. I could almost feel the hormones firing, ratcheting up the pace—and my labour's progress.

I could almost feel the hormones firing!

A couple of times I asked Liliana a question: "The contractions pick up when I walk around, so should I keep walking?" She didn't reply. With a shrug, she simply handed the process back to me. Coaxed me back to myself.

After an hour, the pain accelerated and I needed a hand to hold. It was there. A silent squeeze. Liliana gave no encouragement, no commentary. Words would interrupt me, bring me back to thought when what I needed was this flow. My eyes were closed, but her support was surrounding. I could feel her focus on me—saw through half-shut eyes, that her own were shut too. It was as if she was moving through each contraction with me. So much birth assistance seems to tell the woman to turn away from her pain. But Liliana did the opposite. She helped me move to its centre.

It suddenly felt right to get into the pool. As with every stage, she got me to follow instinct—her trust in me made me trust myself, like a circuit. The pain peaked and I practically pulled Liliana in with me. Just then, the doorbell rang—the midwife had finally appeared. Although she was untrained to do water births it was happening anyway—and Liliana's confidence and experience of water births eased the situation.

It was almost a quarter before three and I'd begun to push. There was no cheering me on, no cautioning me to slow down and pant. "Your body knows how to get the baby out," I could remember Liliana saying on the doula course. And so it seemed. Two pushes, and she was there—my beautiful daughter, Pearl, had arrived.

Water baby

Angela Horn

Early labour

I awoke at around 6.15am on 6 January—my baby's due date, according to my own calculations. When I got up, a small trickle of amniotic fluid ran down my leg. It was watery and clear with white flecks of vernix—not what I expected. For some reason I thought amniotic fluid would be thick, so I spent about half an hour reading pregnancy books to check. I was having contractions every 4-5 minutes from the time I woke up.

I tried to go back to sleep, but found lying down very uncomfortable so I told Graham that he wouldn't be going to work that day, and got up. I tried to eat, thinking that I would need energy to sustain me through labour, but I really didn't feel like eating.

I felt fine and the contractions were no real problem, still coming every four to five minutes or so. They were like the Braxton Hicks contractions I'd had throughout pregnancy, which had been becoming stronger recently. I thought this was pre-labour and that it would probably go on for a day or so as this was my first baby. From stories I'd heard of other natural labours for first babies it was not uncommon for contractions at five-minute intervals to indicate that there was still a long, long time to go, so I didn't think that this was anything to get too excited about.

When a contraction came I leaned forward, standing up, rocked my hips and focused on breathing out slowly and calmly. I'd practised this so often in Active Birth classes that it was second nature. I tried a few contractions sitting, leaning forward on a chair, but found this really uncomfortable. (I felt too restless and needed to be on the move.) So after that I took them standing up, and later kneeling or on all fours. At around 8.30am I phoned the community midwife.

I'd practised this so often, it was second nature

I wonder, in retrospect, if I had been in pre-labour for a while. I had been getting very strong Braxton Hicks contractions for months, but in the last week or so they had got stronger, and I would often have to stop what I was doing because of them. The day before I went into labour (5 January), I did an hour-long aqua-aerobics class. I felt strong contractions whenever I jumped up and down, so I put plenty of energy into the exercises! The aqua-aerobics teacher was pointing at me accusingly, saying: "I can see you're having contractions in my pool! We don't want a water birth *here,* thank you very much!" I think the contractions had been coming every 20 minutes or so for a while but since they only felt strong enough to interrupt my activities if I was doing something, like exercising or walking briskly, I just considered them to be practice for the real thing. Anyway, on 6 January it definitely was the real thing.

I used these early hours of labour to do all the jobs that I wouldn't want to do later—checking my pets and phoning friends. I felt contractions coming on long before they required my full concentration, so I could say "I need to go now" and finish the calls. The activity took my mind off the contractions and I didn't find them difficult to deal with. Some were more intense than others—for the tougher ones I dropped onto all fours and rocked my hips backwards and forwards. When the midwife phoned back I was feeling inexplicably emotional and didn't want to talk to her—I actually cried a little bit, but wasn't really distressed. I wasn't scared at all, just excited. I put the tears down to my hormones, and the emotional patch only lasted about 10 minutes.

The midwife arrives

At around 9.30am the midwife arrived. It was Norma, who I'd met a couple of times before. She was supportive, confident, friendly and very hands-off. We talked and she observed me for a while. Then she offered to do an internal. I had discussed with the midwives previously that I would prefer not to have any internals in labour unless necessary and Norma made it clear that it was entirely up to me whether I wanted to have one or not, but reassured me that she would be gentle and would stop if I wanted, so I was happy for her to go ahead.

I thought that it couldn't be established labour, because it wasn't difficult to cope with, so I was surprised to be told that my cervix was 4-5cm dilated, and that the baby was likely to be born in the early afternoon (it was about 10am at this point). Norma could feel the bag of waters bulging in front of the baby's head, so the fluid I'd seen earlier must have been a hindwater leak. As the baby's head descended it was preventing any more fluid from leaking away and the forewaters were still cushioning its head. The head was 2/5 palpable, i.e. 3/5 engaged; before labour it had been 3/5 palpable for the past six weeks.

Labour can be fun!

I asked Graham to start assembling the birth pool, and found that I needed to devote more effort to dealing with the contractions. I put on some music, turned the lights down and turned on the lava lamp; the Christmas tree was still up, complete with fairy lights, and the whole effect was lovely. I have very fond memories of grooving along to my favourite music, feeling perfectly normal in between contractions and rocking on all fours during them, singing along with the music. Graham needed some help with the pool, so I didn't get to 'groove' for very long.

Norma just chatted and watched me, checking the baby's heart rate and my blood pressure regularly. We were talking about animals, and Norma said "Well, you've seen animals give birth. You know what to do. Just do whatever feels natural to you."

Helping to sort out the pool was a great distraction. Graham and I chatted and worked and it could have been any normal day—except that every few minutes I had to excuse myself and deal with a contraction. Our three cats found the pool very interesting and stood on the side watching the water. One of them fell in! I wasn't worried about the hygiene aspect as the pool came complete with a non-chlorine water sterilising kit and filter.

The contractions got closer and more intense, and by 11.30am I definitely wanted the pool right away, so I got in while it was still filling. This was a good move, as I could direct the hose on my back and tummy during contractions.

Music was playing all the time. Rock and pop songs with rousing choruses (turned up loud during contractions) which I could sing along to were my main form of pain relief. I didn't need pethidine—Jimi Hendrix and Abba were quite effective and had few side-effects! I am normally very self-conscious about singing when anyone can hear me because I've been told so often that I have an absolutely dreadful singing voice. However, I was completely uninhibited about singing when in labour and also about making noises later on.

How the pool helped

The pool was a great help. Although it didn't take the pain away, it was warm and soothing and I certainly found it easier to cope with contractions *in* the pool than *out*. The support of the water made it very easy for me to switch quickly between positions—I had to be on all fours for contractions but between them I was floating, squatting, sitting or standing. Squatting positions were far easier to hold than on land. Sometimes I went completely under the water during or between contractions. It was very relaxing to feel surrounded by warm water and to feel quite alone in this peaceful place. The water helped me to focus on breathing out slowly too. Breathing out under water, or with just my mouth under the water, I could blow bubbles and watch and hear the breath, as opposed to just feeling it. It was a rhythmic process and a good distraction during contractions—duck under the water, breathe out slowly, surface and breathe in and then duck under again.

During some moderate contractions I tried wearing a snorkel and staying underwater for the whole contraction. This was quite fun at first, but having the mask on my face got a bit annoying later. Sometimes I kept my head above the water and sang or made other sounds as I breathed out. When things got really intense I hummed and vocalised in other ways, again as practised in the Active Birth classes. When I could have cried out in pain, I hummed "Ommmmmm" during the out-breath. It's not that I attribute any special qualities to that particular word, but it was a convenient sound to make, and it helped a lot. I thought that crying out would not be helpful... It would make me more tense and might make those around me tense.

I put some Lavender and clary sage essential oils in the water. Regardless of whether they help labour, they smell nice and it was relaxing to be surrounded by fragrance rising from the surface of the warm pool.

Water temperature

The water temperature was around 34 degrees centigrade for the first stage—any hotter and I think I'd have felt sick. During the second stage I would have liked it to be warmer, but I was too preoccupied to ask or to do anything about it. Next time I would try to remember.

Norma recorded the water temperature at intervals, and asked if I was comfortable. Characteristically, she was focusing upon what would make me feel good, rather than trying to tell me what temperature the pool should be. Don't let anyone try to tell you what temperature the pool should be; as long as you are not overheating during labour (which would make you very uncomfortable) and your baby is not hanging around in cold water after birth, all that matters is that the temperature is right for the mother.

I got out of the pool a few times to go to the loo—I knew that pee was sterile so it was OK to go in the pool and, let's face it, a cat had already fallen in there so I could hardly get fussy about water hygiene! However, I also knew that it was good to move around as much as possible and that the process of climbing in and out of the pool involved major leg-raises and hip-hitching that would help the baby to move down. Contractions outside the water were far harder to cope with.

The hard work starts..

As my labour progressed I felt sharp pains in my hips and the all-fours position became vital to take the pressure off my sacrum. Graham rubbed my back during contractions and kept me supplied with drinks of hot water with honey and lemon juice. I needed to have Graham there... I missed him when he left the room. He was very calm—we all were—and very involved in the labour. In fact, I had far more physical contact with Graham than I did with the midwife.

Norma seemed instinctively to know that I wanted to be touched as little as possible and that I did not need her to 'deliver' the baby but just to check that the baby and I were both well, while I got on with the job of giving birth.

During what was probably transition the contractions were very intense and close together and overwhelming, but I felt dreamy. I still felt the pain, yet seemed able to fit a lot of rest into the minute between contractions. My body's natural pain-managing mechanisms were working well. Although dreamy, I was still rational, still myself. I felt quite romantic during this 'dreamy' time and kept looking at Graham and thinking soppy things, like how much I loved him and how wonderful it was that I was having our baby.

Suddenly, I felt wide awake and perfectly lucid so I asked Norma if I was in transition. She said that normally people got very ratty in transition—I'd not been at all ratty so far. (In fact, I was probably more polite than I am usually.) Norma offered to do an internal if I wanted to find out but I thought that either I was or I wasn't in transition and an internal wouldn't change the fact, so why bother?

Anyway, it turned out that I must have been because, during a very hard contraction, I felt the waters break—fluid gushed out under pressure, and Norma said the cervix was probably totally drawn up.

Nearly there...

At one point I decided to get out of the pool and walk around to help the baby descend. Having told everyone that I was going to get out for a little while, I stood up and then a contraction came. My precise words were "Stuff this for a game of soldiers!" I went straight back in the water, and didn't get out again until the baby was born!

When I felt the urge to push, things became primal. Low, bellowing, moose-like noises came out as I pushed. It was like vomiting—huge convulsions over which I had minimal control.

Norma said that when the head crowned, I should push it out however felt natural and bring the baby to the surface in my own way. Crowning seemed to be a long way off when she said this. I poked a finger inside and the head felt like a lump of spongy meat. I wasn't sure that it was a head at all but what else could it be? I remembered my antenatal class teacher saying that the head would not feel like a head at this stage because of molding and was reassured.

The head crowned around 15 minutes later. The burning sensation was intense, and I thought "Aha! This is what they mean by the 'ring of fire'!" but it didn't matter because I knew the baby would be born very soon. I was kneeling upright with my knees wide apart so gravity was able to do a lot to stop the head receding. I remember instinctively making small movements to give the baby more space to come out. At this stage I was very alert and was giving a running commentary on what the baby's head was doing because there was no way anyone outside the pool could see what was going on.

I realised that I could make voluntary pushes between contractions and that they really did move things down. I knew that voluntary pushing was A Bad Thing but, hey, it could still get results! "Norma, I can push in between contractions. Shall I?" "No!" came the reply, "there's no point in pushing in between contractions. Just wait for the contractions to do the work." Huh—no official sanction. I pushed anyway when I thought she wasn't looking.

With a huge push and a contraction, the baby's head was born. I felt around his neck to check that the cord wasn't around it. The baby's body was firmly clamped inside—there was no way this one was going to just slither out. I waited for the next contraction. (It felt like at least 10 minutes but according to my notes it was only one minute.) And then I thought "Sod it!" and gave a huge shove anyway, but there was probably a contraction there too. The baby's shoulders, arms and chest were born but he was *still* stuck fast again at the tummy. (If I'd been on my back this might have been a case of shoulder dystocia, by the way.) I thought, "Stuff this. I'm not waiting for another contraction" so I grabbed hold of the baby under the arms, gave a big push and pulled the rest of him out.

I thought "Sod it!" and gave a shove anyway

I brought the baby to the surface. He gave a huge yell and turned bright red, and I was amazed to see that it was a boy—Lee. We had been convinced that it was a girl. Then I noticed the midwives saying things like "Look at the size of that!" and, ominously, directed at the baby: "I dread to think what you've done to that perineum". He was big and strong, very solid, covered in vernix and obviously vigorous.

I climbed out of the pool, holding him close to me, and sat on the bed next to Graham. The baby was covered in a towel, but with his skin bare next to mine. I offered him my breast. He wasn't very interested in sucking but he made an attempt. It was a great relief to sit down after nine hours on my feet and knees. I felt perfectly normal, if a little tired. I certainly didn't experience the post-delivery euphoria that many women have, even though it was a great birth in perfect surroundings. I felt very business-like about it and, being English, I just wanted a cup of tea! I cuddled Lee and comforted him—he didn't cry for long, just briefly at the initial shock of being born—and we waited for the cord to stop pulsating so that he had his natural quota of blood. After about 15 minutes there was no detectable pulse in the cord so Graham clamped and cut it. No one had touched our son apart from us for these first minutes of his life. No one handled him roughly, stuck tubes in his nose or mouth to suction them, put him down on cold surfaces, or subjected him to any 'standard procedures'. They weren't necessary. All he needed was a cuddle and the warmth of his mother's body.

The third stage

I had a natural third stage but the placenta took an hour to turn up. Norma wasn't worried about the time as there was just one large gush of blood and clots, then very little blood loss. I think the placenta was sitting there, waiting for me to push it out. I could have done with more direction here but both midwives were busy with the baby and paperwork. I did feel slightly abandoned but I guess I should have asked for help. Lee was in excellent shape and was huge: 4.25kg, 9lb 6oz.

I had a second-degree tear straight down the midline, which didn't need to be stitched as it wasn't bleeding. Perhaps if I'd resisted that voluntary pushing I could have avoided the tear. Norma commented that being in the pool would have helped to minimise tearing. (Like having a hot compress *in situ*, it provides warm counter-pressure against the perineum). I lost at least 500ml (just over 1 pint) of blood. That was what made it to the measuring jug but there was plenty that landed elsewhere. I was healthy, my blood pressure was fine, I didn't feel faint or even unwell and blood tests three days later showed that I wasn't anaemic.

When everything was over I felt absolutely fine—tired, but not exhausted, and very happy. That night the three of us slept together, Lee curled up against me in the most secure and natural way for a baby to sleep.

Conclusions

I would do it all again just the same way... tomorrow! It took nine hours to deliver Lee, including a second stage of about 1 hour 15 minutes. It might seem that I was lucky but it took a full 13 months of careful preparation— exercise and research—to help luck produce the goods! Of course, there are some eventualities that you cannot prepare for but there are others which you *can* do something about. Perhaps preparing for those things I *could* do something about stopped me worrying about the factors I *couldn't* control.

If there had been some complication and transfer to hospital had become necessary, it would have helped me to know that I'd done just about everything I could to have a normal labour and birth and that if intervention was necessary in spite of all that preparation and my best efforts, then I would be very glad that it was available.

The midwifery care I received was excellent. Throughout my pregnancy the community midwives I saw were all supportive of homebirth and seemed confident and well informed on the subject.

During the labour, although I found that I did not want to be fussed over, it gave me confidence to see that Norma was so calm and relaxed. The impression I got from her throughout was that she was perfectly sure that this labour was going to progress smoothly and I felt that if she was so confident, with all her experience, then I certainly didn't have anything to worry about. Having said that, if there had been a problem then I have no doubt that she would have been well prepared to deal with it—and I would have trusted her and accepted her recommendations. Thank you, Norma!

Finally, some tips for using a birth pool... (from Sylvie)

- ♥ Put the pool up before labour starts so you know how it fits together
- ♥ Make sure the immersion is switched on, in case extra hot water is needed
- ♥ Get a big sponge or foam pad, or a folded towel, for kneeling on underwater
- ♥ Place a large tarpaulin under the pool for worry-free splashing and dripping
- ♥ Don't immerse yourself in water (of any kind—bath or birthing pool) until you're at least 5cm dilated. When your labour has progressed to that stage, you'll be having contractions thick and fast (perhaps one minute apart).
- ♥ Lean forward at all times. This is not a time for lying back and relaxing. The baby needs oxygen and its supply might be affected if you recline.
- ♥ Don't have the water too hot. Heat can be dangerous for an unborn baby.
- ♥ If contractions become weaker or less frequent, get out straight away. It's likely you've got in too soon. If, after an hour and a half or so in the water, nothing seems to have happened, seek advice from a professional.
- ♥ If you prefer to avoid the hassle of a birthing pool, consider using an ordinary warm bath if only for a few moments late on in labour. This will soften your perineum, which will be able to stretch more easily for the birth.

Unscripted reality show

Ruth Clark

The players: Me—Ruth
Adam—my husband
Ben—the star player
Eddy—our 2-year-old son
Sue—my midwife
Julie—my other midwife
Maggie—supporter for Ruth and Adam
Kerry—supporter for Eddy
Daniel—supporter for Eddy and also my brother

My first birth experience hadn't been as I had hoped. Due to a premature footling breech my plans for a home birth had been well and truly ruined. So this time round I was twice as determined to have my baby at home. I was delighted when I discovered the baby was cephalic (head-down), a perfect LOA [left occiput anterior], i.e. with its back round to the left side of my bump) and I was ecstatic once we got past that magical 37 weeks [after which point NHS midwives will cover a home birth]. I was really excited about going into labour, no worries about anything... This was going to be good and everything that my last labour wasn't. My NHS midwives were supportive and we got on really well.

I was woken on 15 January at 5.00am by Eddy, who was crying. As I went in to see him I noticed a slight discomfort in my lower abdomen that was coming and going, I put this down to wind. After dealing with Eddy I went back to bed and listened to him singing and talking to himself until he went back to sleep at 6.15. All this time I was aware of the abdominal discomfort, only slight, but enough to keep me awake. (I am a light sleeper.)

At 6.30 I decided that I needed to open my bowels. I thought I would feel better after this but I didn't. If anything, I felt slightly worse. I wondered if, as this was six days before my due date, these were contractions and decided that if they were, they must be Braxton Hicks.

At 7.00am I got up and fed the cats (all seven of them). The contractions were now coming about every 10 minutes and were getting stronger and longer but were easily bearable—I just breathed through them. I now also noticed a lower back pain but still did not think that I was in labour.

At 7.15am I needed the toilet again, this time it was much looser and I noticed a show. I wondered if this was the real thing as there were now four signs but I was not convinced.

At 7.30am I thought that maybe I should wake Adam. I told him I thought that I might be in labour. He said "OK" and asked if I needed him, and then he went back to sleep. I decided I'd better phone the other people who were due to come over. Kerry had just arrived home from working a night shift and she had taken a sleeping tablet and was about to go to bed; she was not going to miss this for the world and set out to walk across town to our house. Daniel was on his way to work so I couldn't get hold of him. Maggie did not answer her phone (it was broken), so I phoned her partner's mobile. He was halfway across the country but managed to get a message to Maggie via relatives who live nearby. I got hold of Daniel at 7.55am. I told him there was no rush as he wanted to go elsewhere on the way.

By 8.00am Adam was getting out of bed. I saw him naked at the top of the stairs and through bleary eyes he told me he needed to go to the toilet. I told him in no uncertain terms "I need to go first." And once again I opened my bowels. My contractions were now very close together.

At 8.05am, still sitting on the toilet, I had the first really intense contraction. It was very different to the previous ones, which had all been really low down and opening-out type contractions. This one was from the top of my uterus, a really strong pushing contraction. My first thought was that this shouldn't be happening yet, I couldn't possibly be at this part of my labour as I hadn't had the painful bit yet. However my body was pushing and there was nothing I could do that was going to stop it. I then decided that I needed to do my hair (which is down to my waist), so I unplaited it and asked Adam for my hairbrush. I also decided that I needed my TENS machine on; it was far too late for this but it seemed the right thing to do at the time.

After two or three more contractions I put my hand down between my legs and could feel something sticking out! I lifted myself off the toilet seat and asked Adam what it was... it was the amniotic membranes bulging out and was about the size of a grapefruit. At this point I decided that I needed a midwife rather urgently. She was the one person that I had omitted to phone when I made my calls earlier so she didn't even know I was in labour.

Adam went downstairs and called the labour hotline. He asked to speak to Sue. The person on the other end told him that she was a community midwife and he would have to call their office. He came back up to me moaning about this and how useless they were. "Did you tell them that I am in labour?"... "Oh... no". He went back downstairs and tried again.

At 8.25am Sue phoned back. She heard me shout out at the next contraction and suggested to Adam that he should be upstairs with me. I then shouted down that I could feel the baby's head. Sue said that she would phone back in two minutes once Adam had put the phone on the extension upstairs.

I instinctively kept my hand on the baby's head from when I first felt it. The next contraction came and the head moved out a bit and then back in again. Adam brought the phone upstairs and began to spread a groundsheet on the floor so that I could get off the toilet. As he finished doing this I had another contraction. With this one my waters broke, out came the baby's head, followed by his body. As I delivered my baby I lifted myself off the toilet seat, brought him up between my legs and cradled our second son in my arms as I sat back down again. Adam looked round and folded the groundsheet back up again. Then the phone rang: it was Maggie. Adam asked her the time, so we now knew our new son had been born at 8.30am. Almost immediately the phone buzzed again. It was Sue, expecting to talk Adam through the birth. He just said "Listen!" She heard the cries and asked if we were OK. She also asked if we wanted to call an ambulance or just wait until she got there. As we were fine we said we would wait and she said that she would get there as soon as possible. I offered baby my breast but he nuzzled at my nipple for a bit and then went to sleep.

At 8.35am Eddy appeared in the bathroom doorway. He looked at me sitting on the toilet and said "Baby!" and then came to join us. Adam got a big towel to wrap around baby and me to keep us warm and then decided that he'd better get some clothes on before everyone arrived; he'd had no time to dress up to this point and I had been wearing his bathrobe. I then asked Adam to take some photos while the cord was still intact. Kerry arrived first and took some photos of all four of us. She then looked after Eddy.

At 9.00am Julie arrived. She had got dressed in the dark in a hurry and was wearing pink socks with her dark blue uniform and she had also been stopped by the police for speeding on her way to me. (They let her go as soon as she explained the situation.) As the cord had stopped pulsating, I was happy for her to clamp it and Adam cut it. Baby was then wrapped in another towel and Adam had his first cuddle while Julie helped me off the toilet and onto the floor. Adam then put baby on the floor so that I could lean against him while the placenta was born. While I was waiting for the placenta I noticed my window cleaner cleaning the bathroom window! At 9.10 I had a contraction and felt the placenta move down. Two minutes later I had another smaller one with which the placenta was born. Julie examined me and told me that I had sustained a small tear, which I decided not to have stitched. I stayed sitting on the floor while baby was checked and weighed. He was 7lb 12oz.

By this time Daniel, Maggie and Sue had arrived. Sue was later than she had hoped because she had skidded on ice and put her car into a ditch. At some point another midwife arrived but I have no idea who she was and she left once Sue got there. Maggie ran a bath for me and made drinks for everyone. Adam stood on our back doorstep to have a cigarette and shook a bit—poor chap still hadn't been to the toilet. I took baby into the bath with me where he had his first breastfeed for about 20 minutes. Eddy kept coming up to check on us and to look at his new brother.

I was then dispatched to my bed, even though I felt full of energy and not the least bit tired. I wanted to tell the whole world what a wonderful experience I'd just had; it was a total contrast to Eddy's birth. I was far too energetic and high to sleep, so Adam brought me the phone so that I could call all our friends and family to tell them the news.

It really was the most wonderful and empowering experience of my whole life. I thoroughly enjoyed my labour and birth and I wasn't the least bit worried or frightened about birthing my baby without a midwife in attendance. It was so natural and instinctive. All we needed now was a name for our son. One helpful friend suggested Lou! Eddy offered Mr McGregor (he's a big Peter Rabbit fan). Our baby was three days old when we decided to call him Ben.

It was just like he said it would be

Rachel Urbach

I gave birth at home, at age 38, in water without using any drugs. My [identical] twin sister had had a baby the previous year, with the usual story of failed home delivery due to minor complications followed by the cascade of interventions at hospital ending in a caesarean.

I read Michel Odent's book *Birth Reborn* and was inspired at the stories of healthy births—the fact that he finally avoided the use of chemical pain relief altogether because it seemed to interfere with the natural pain-relieving processes of the body. I searched widely for a sympathetic midwife and was so lucky to eventually find one, who visited me at home and helped my confidence. I think state of mind is so important. I also did some hypnosis, or visualisation of the birthing process, which I think helped.

My baby was born after a nine-hour labour. To my amazement, it was like Michel described—I became almost like an animal, or went into another level of consciousness beyond pain. The part I remember as the most difficult was the beginning—moments of fear—then gaining confidence—more moments of fear—reassurance from the midwife—then feeling like a fish in water being thrown about by the contractions and finally roaring as she came out, not with pain (as is so often the stereotype we see of labouring women) but with power.

It left me feeling so proud of my body.

You're a mammal!

Michel Odent

A week ago on Sunday, I was at a conference in California. I was a keynote speaker. My topic was provocative. It was why and how we should dehumanise childbirth. There were two organisers, two midwives, Iona and Laura. Iona was pregnant and due quite soon—this month—and expecting her first baby. Laura, who herself had three children, was at the same time Iona's partner as a practising midwife, and also her midwife for this birth.

Iona introduced me on Saturday at about 11.30am and while I was speaking some people noticed that she was often touching her back. Then at about 3.00pm she had a rupture of membranes at the conference. So she went back home, which was about 20 minutes from there, with Laura. Luckily there was a third midwife involved in the organisation of the conference.

In the end, real labour started in the middle of the night and Iona gave birth on Sunday morning exactly a week ago. And I just heard before leaving (because I left on Sunday afternoon) that she had had a baby boy. But I called her yesterday to find out more. She told me an interesting story.

She told me there was a time when many women—when the baby was not far away—used to say "Do something! I can't do it. I can't do it!" But Laura told her "You can do it. You're a mammal!" Because of my lecture they had changed their approach. Originally, Iona had planned to give birth in front of some television cameras but then she heard me talking about privacy and cameras. I'd also said that it was important to be careful about the presence of the baby's father. So in the end she had much more privacy than she'd expected to have. It was her first baby and it was wonderful. And Laura had said twice "You can do it! You're a mammal!"

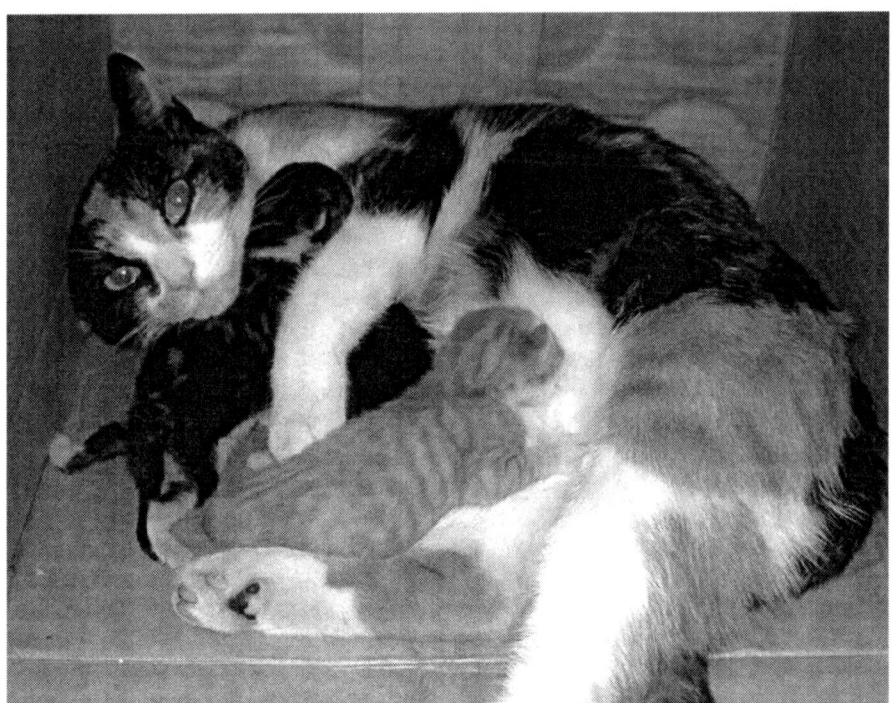

Other mammals are usually very good at seeking out privacy and just getting on with it...

Who needs pain?

Sue Pakes

I always enjoyed the conversations at playgroups when they invariably came round to the subject of childbirth, a bit like discussing exam results when you know you've done well! It seems that I have been one of the lucky ones and, yes, it does happen.

As the due date of my first child loomed, my mother did admit that she had not had too much trouble giving birth to my three siblings and myself, though you don't know how much gets forgotten over time. In those days it was customary to have the first child in hospital and any further births at home, so in the back of my mind I felt confident that if we had more than one child, I too could enjoy a home delivery. Also, I felt that at long last my wide hips may be coming into their own!

The delivery of your first baby is certainly a surprise. Nothing can prepare you for what is going to happen. I was well planned for the event: I had given up work six weeks before, had rested at home, spent sessions at the local swimming pool building up my stamina, requested a water birth at the hospital and had even spent time taping my favourite music ready for the hours I expected to be in labour.

When the time arrived, not even knowing that I was in labour but wondering why I had been sick and why was I suffering from what I thought to be bad period pains, we drove to the maternity hospital. On arrival at around 6.00am, I was examined by a midwife. To her surprise, she found that I was sufficiently dilated to move to a delivery suite. Once we were there and I had climbed onto the bed, she went in search of pain relief. Within minutes, however, my waters had gone and I was ready to push! As my husband called for someone 'quickly', I couldn't believe that it was all happening so fast. There wasn't sufficient time for any pethidine, so I was offered gas and air. When the moment came to push I pushed as hard as I could and, after a short amount of pain, our son was born at 7.10am weighing in at 8lb 8oz—and I didn't even need any stitches.

So when it came to the due date of our second child, I wondered if I would have a similar easy delivery. Again, things seemed to get going early in the morning (after a good night's sleep) and I awoke again to uncomfortable period pains. I was adamant that I was going to have a shower before the midwife arrived to assess me and even managed to wash my hair! In the meantime, slightly apprehensively, my husband called the midwife at 6.30am. When she arrived around 7.20am and asked me to lie down on the bed, I knew that as soon as I lay down I wouldn't be going anywhere. Again, after one massive push our daughter was born at 7.42am, weighing in at 9lb 8oz. Throughout the time, I had been totally calm and when I saw how relaxed the midwife was, I felt I too had little to worry about. My body took over.

Husband takes charge

Alan Low

We had returned late on the Saturday night from a friend's wedding reception and climbed into bed, with me still feeling the effects of an over-indulgence of food and alcohol. Sleep came upon me with ease until I was rudely awakened by a sharp dig in the ribs by Karen, my beloved, who rather nervously announced that she thought it had started. Being a loving, sensitive and supportive partner, my immediate response was to enquire: "Have you had a show yet? No?! Well go back to sleep and don't wake me until you have." Could this really have been Mr Sensitive talking or was it the booze and lack of sleep taking over? (That's my excuse and I'm sticking to it!) A slightly more aggressive dig in the ribs followed and was accompanied by a short, sharp volley of verbal abuse and threatening behaviour. I was stung into action, so crawled out of bed and attempted to look sharp and alert, ready for anything, but in reality of course was a total wreck and looked it—no fooling anyone.

> Could this really have been Mr Sensitive talking or was it the booze and lack of sleep taking over?

We agreed that we should keep busy, so tidied the house, had a bath, played Scrabble (I won) and before we knew it 3.00am turned into 7.00am. It was now time to call Liz, who had helped and advised us so far and was our 'expert'. She had agreed to help out and had three children of her own, two of which had been born at home. I collected Liz around 9.00am and returned to find that the contractions were regular enough to warrant calling the midwife.

In the months leading up to the birth we had some difficulties (understatement) with 'The Establishment' regarding our desire for a home birth, with a few midwives vehemently opposed. We had expressed our discontent to the local Head of Midwifery, who had agreed that the attending midwife would not be one of the dissenters. Unfortunately, on that fateful morn, No.1 choice was ill, No.2 had a day off, No.3 was Head Dissenter (didn't even bother calling her, she would have been out on her broomstick anyway) but No.4 answered. Great! Or so we thought. Much to our surprise, Karen was answered with a torrent of abuse for choosing a home birth and for also politely refusing the midwife's offer of having a student in attendance. She said she would be around soon, but was not happy.

> The effect was the contractions stopped completely

The effect of this event was to stop the contractions completely, but normal service resumed 20 minutes later. We discussed and collectively agreed that this lady was not for us. Karen and Liz agreed that I would turn her away at the door while they hid—thanks. Time for my cool, calm approach towards problem-solving to surface. I took control and phoned the hospital to find out the alternatives and demand action. All they could suggest was to make the peace with Midwife No.4, as she was all that was available—time for Mr Cool to panic. "We can do it ourselves!" I proudly announced. "Boil some water and fetch towels!" Liz calmed the hysteria by informing us that this was illegal and that she would contact her ex-midwife and now friend, Jo, who was a practising independent midwife. She agreed to come but would have to obtain the appropriate approvals from the State Health Authority first. This was to be a momentous obstacle but she managed to battle through OK and arrived on our doorstep at 1pm—phew! The next stop was to provide her with some assistance and back-up, courtesy of Jan, who we all knew and was an ex-nurse and current antenatal teacher.

The first examination revealed, much to everyone's amazement, that Karen was 8cm dilated. Around 2.00pm the second stage commenced, a time Karen had been dreading, but Jo reassured her by saying that whilst it would probably be painful it shouldn't take too long as she was doing so well. 'Too long' to someone (like me) in intense pain would be 10 seconds.

'Not too long' lasted two hours for Karen

'Not too long' lasted two hours for Karen, who was by this time starting to tire. Digby (the silly name we had christened the bump once the scan had revealed our baby was to be a boy) started to crown, but a further 25 minutes passed. Jo and Jan constantly reassured Karen that 'one more push will do it' but none of us really believed it until suddenly, without warning, Digby shot out and was fantastically caught one-handed by Jo.

On closer examination Digby appeared to be woefully short of a few vital attributes that would make his position as the rightful Captain of the England football team difficult to attain. Digby's attributes were more suited for netball so I found myself wiping the tears of joy away, holding our beautiful daughter, while the third stage commenced. I looked at her and thought, "Just like her mother—late!" It made me want to weep!

Meanwhile, back at the action, Karen had finished the third stage relatively quickly but was haemorrhaging badly, was very pale and was starting to shake uncontrollably as she was going into shock. The scene started to resemble an out-take from *The Exorcist* but, fortunately, Jo and Jan quickly averted any danger and the bleeding subsided.

At the first available moment I dashed downstairs to crack the champagne and returned to find the new mum feeding our daughter, which immediately restored the lump in my throat and dampness to my eyes. By 9.30pm, everyone had left and we were left alone in total amazement looking at the little bundle laid between us. Our first sleepless night was soon to be upon us...

But I thought you'd be there!

Sylvie Donna

I look back on my second child's birth with a great feeling of peace, happiness and even wonder. Nina-Jay was born on 15 December at 11.30 in the evening, just two hours after I experienced the first contraction; the placenta came out painlessly with another contraction, a few moments later. Her Apgar score was 10 and she weighed in at a very healthy weight. There was no problem with blood loss and no need for any stitching—I only had a little superficial tearing, which healed in a couple of days. I started breastfeeding my new baby moments after she was born and we continued—with breaks!—until she was nearly 2 years old, without any problems.

In the three weeks before the evening of her birth I had experienced numerous painless or low-pain contractions. The contractions which started at 9.30pm on her 'birth day', while I was doing the washing up, came on very suddenly. They were much stronger than any I had felt in the days and weeks before. In fact, they were completely absorbing. I was immediately on my hands and knees on the kitchen floor.

Fortunately, Michel Odent, my caregiver for this birth, was already in the house when these contractions started so there was no problem with this being a short labour. Just before I'd started doing the washing up, he and I had sat at the kitchen table after an enormous dinner, talking about my life and all my problems and I realise that something in me had relaxed during that conversation. I'd been worried about the future but Michel had somehow reassured me. The day before this, I had called him, thinking I was in labour, and had had to apologise when he arrived since my contractions had stopped. He decided to stay at our place that night and in the morning said he would like to come to dinner again later that day and again stay overnight. (We were living a long way from his home in London.) I must say, I wasn't keen when he said this because I had visions of cooking for him and apologising for the next two weeks—but it turned out that he was right to return so soon. When he arrived at around 4.00pm, I was fast asleep, having had a huge and wonderful lunchtime curry. My partner was at home that day because of a quirk in his timetable, so I hadn't needed to look after 2-year-old Anjula—I could rest.

With these sudden, overwhelmingly powerful contractions, I soon felt the need to stagger upstairs and start some sonorous groaning. Michel, hearing the noise, emerged from the room we'd assigned him—next door to the bathroom, where I was—and asked if he could please check the baby's heartbeat and position. His brief examination reassured him that conditions were ideal for me to labour undisturbed. Firstly, palpation of my bump had told him I had a full bag of waters. This meant there was little danger of the umbilical cord prolapsing or becoming compressed.

Secondly, he established that the position of my baby was fine—LOA—left occiput anterior. This is the best possible position and a common one if the woman hasn't been in the habit of leaning back and 'putting her feet up' during pregnancy! (Later Michel told me his 'treatment'—i.e. to leave me to labour undisturbed—would not have been different if she had also been in a posterior position, like her big sister. He said he has found that women find better positions for helping the baby turn if left alone, undisturbed.) Thirdly, Michel confirmed with a fetal stethoscope (a Pinard, which is a tapered tube shape) that the fetal heartbeat was strong. He was also reassured to see that on my return to the bathroom I was spontaneously labouring in favourable positions— leaning forward, either standing, on my hands and knees, or on my knees in front of the toilet when I was throwing up! He knew this would mean avoiding compressing the vena cava, which would happen lying down, and which is important for the baby's oxygen supply. While I laboured alone, in peace, Michel waited and listened from the room next door. He even waited outside while I gave birth.

Phil, my partner, helped me throughout my brief two-hour labour. As each contraction ripped into me I fully understood why some women choose drug-based pain relief or a caesarean—but I knew I must not even mention any of these thoughts out loud. A few contractions into my labour I said to Phil "Two children are enough! We really don't need to have a third one, you know." Wisely ignoring my comment, he ran up and down the stairs fetching things for me—candles for candlelight, something to tie my hair back... (We'd agreed he'd do this in advance.) Meanwhile, Michel continued to keep watch from the next room, without making himself seen. He knew from long experience that the best support would be to leave me completely undisturbed, with a feeling of being unobserved. The sounds I made would be enough to tell him if all was going well. Of course, he administered no drugs and insisted on no routines. Nature had her own routines in mind...

Then, within two hours of feeling that first contraction, I gave birth. Moments before, Anjula had woken up so Phil had had to go and console her. After sitting on the toilet for a few minutes, straining to do a non-existent poo, I suddenly stood up, lifted up my arms, flexed my knees slightly and gave birth! Between my feet, bundled up in a large ball, was a plastic sheet which I'd been 'relocating' around the house in a preoccupied manner for the few days before I went into labour. So much strength was coursing through my body when I was ready to give birth that I didn't need anyone's help or support. I thought about various things I'd read... I thought of Inuit (Eskimos)—supporting their wives from behind and pushing down on the bump so as to help the baby, and I focused in on my own baby within me. Then I thought, "Baby, be born!"—calm, joyful words which passed through my head quite spontaneously. Then suddenly, I gave two wonderful strong, clear, purposeful painfree pushes. The ring of fire I then felt made me consciously realise my new baby's head must have crowned.

I momentarily felt worried I would tear. Then, thinking "Oh, I don't care if I rip in two," I flicked my hips forward. Reaching down to feel what was going on, I was shocked to feel a head. "Michel!" I shouted, anxious that I should be giving birth without his help. Knowing it would be dangerous to disturb me at this point, he ignored me and carried on simply silently watching through the crack in the door. There was a moment's pause, then again I flicked my hips forwards. In a sudden gush my baby was born and, confused, I felt another gush seconds later.

I looked down, transfixed for what must have been only a few seconds, admiring my new baby's features. Suddenly she let out a cry and saying, "Don't cry," I took her up in my arms and instinctively put her to my breast.

There was none of the hesitation I'd expected to feel. Having read about so many problem situations, I had wondered whether breastfeeding would be so easy the second time around. My new baby sucked as if for the thousandth time, not the first. As I looked down it dawned on me that the second gush had been the placenta... It was all so fast! Beautifully alert, my baby was gazing quizzically into my eyes as she breastfed. Michel came in at this point and was reassured to see the placenta lying by my side, born and whole, a sign that all was properly finished and safe. My husband was sad to have missed the birth and 2-year-old Anjula, who'd just woken up, looked amazed at her mother holding a new baby in her arms.

It was wonderful not having someone else 'catch' the baby for me. It was also wonderful being able to discover her sex myself and pick her up for the first time without anyone observing or 'checking' on me. The most wonderful aspect of this birth, though, was the feeling of strength I had. I felt so strong, both physically and mentally. I didn't need anyone to support me as I suddenly stood up, swung round, raised my arms in the air, elbows bent, feet planted firmly on the floor some distance apart, knees flexed. I certainly didn't need anyone to tell me I was fully dilated. Somewhere deep inside, I knew it was time to push. The feeling of pushing—two long, clear, happy pushes—was very positive and also completely painless, as I said before. The ring of fire which I immediately became aware of at the end of these pushes was also not painful or 'weak-feeling'. There was never any need to 'pant' or control my breathing—I just felt poised, focused, very alert and decisive. And I was strong physically in the sense that I had no problems with low blood pressure and no feelings of weakness after the birth. This had been a truly authentic fetus ejection reflex.

After this birth, and my third a couple of years later, I realised again the enormous advantages postnatally of giving birth like this. I understood on a very deep level how *healthy* this type of birth is, physically and psychologically and how little pain there was overall. Most importantly, I saw the advantages for my babies, who were alert, breastfed easily, and who absolutely *thrived*.

Afterwards, I realised how healthy this type of birth is

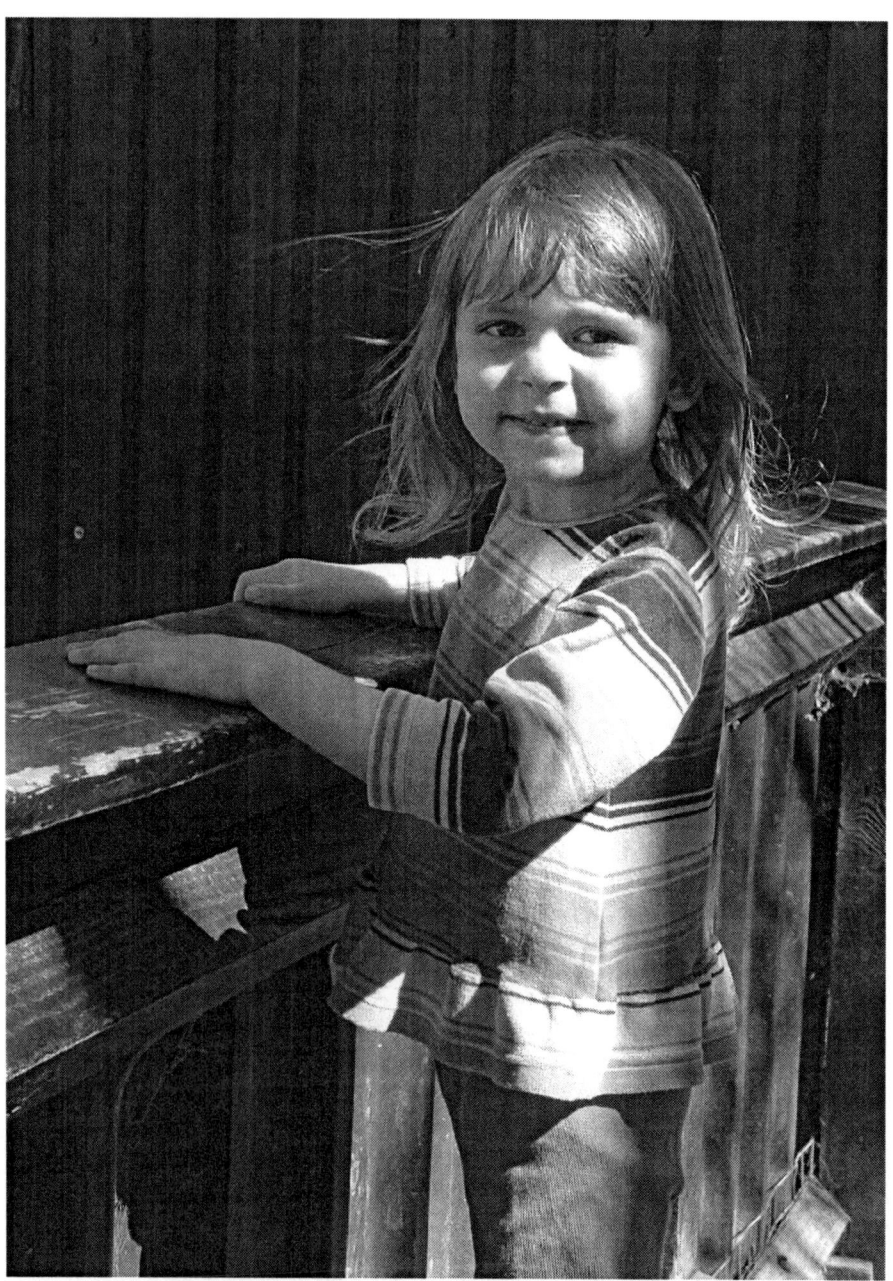

Nina-Jay, aged 3, who was born after a two-hour undisturbed labour, by 'fetus ejection reflex'. This long-forgotten human reflex urgently needs to be rediscovered!

Everything possible for an amazing outcome!

Steve and Olga Mellor

Towards the end of April I was out shopping for some new shoes when my mobile phone buzzed. It was Olga (my Russian fiancée) calling with a big surprise. It seems our last visit together had been more productive than either of us thought. Yes, she was pregnant and we were going to have our first baby. So within one year I went from being single to finding my life partner and expecting my first child.

Because of the visa processing time I was not around for the first few months of the pregnancy as Olga was still in Moscow. It was hard for both of us as we did not get to celebrate like most couples but what we did do was start the process of preparing for our child coming into the world. This is where it got a little interesting.

It was by no means anything like the Cold War of our two nations but, because of our different life experiences, our ideas about how to have a baby differed. Myself, having been born and raised in America, knew exactly how to have a baby: you get pregnant, wait nine months and then go to the hospital where the doctor can give drugs to get through the pain and then he delivers it.

Olga had a completely different plan. Having been raised in Russia and not always having faith in the medical system, she didn't want to have a hospital birth. She wanted to have a home birth, as did many of her friends, with no medication, as she understood that any drug she took, the baby would receive 10 times as strong.

Now I had neighbours years earlier who had had a home birth and at the time I had thought, "How interesting", but I had never thought to myself, "Yes, that is what I want." So Olga wanted to have a home birth and I knew nothing about it. One of my good friends, who was a chiropractor and who had studied a lot about natural ways to heal the body, gave me a book on natural childbirth. So I read the book cover to cover and learnt all I could. The book had me questioning a lot of the traditional things I had heard about giving birth or had seen in films or on TV, when they were showing a woman having a baby. At the same time Olga was attending a series of classes in Moscow, where the main idea was to do everything as naturally as possible, without any interference.

Olga's classes were great as she was not only learning how to deliver, but also talking about birth on a physical, emotional and spiritual level—something I think is missing in the typical American system. So as she would tell me about the classes I would think to myself that some of the stuff she was learning was crazy. But then I would do some more research and find out for myself that it wasn't really. I remember our first conversation about having a home birth. I was scared of the possibility of things going wrong.

I was scared that things would go wrong

And then I would find statistics stating that most C-sections were done on Fridays—wouldn't want to ruin the doctor's weekend!—and that women were actually scheduling their C-sections before they even gave a regular birth a try. It started to appear to me that the medical system seemed just as crazy.

There were many other questions that I found myself asking. Olga didn't want to have any ultrasound scans and that again concerned me. Then I started to ask around to find out the purpose of doing them. No one could really give me a good reason. I heard things like: "To know the baby's sex", "To help predict the due date" or "To find out if the baby is healthy".

But then I would also find out that even though they could find some things out, in most cases there was nothing that could be done. I further learnt that there have been cases of couples who, learning about some defect, chose to abort the pregnancy, only to find out afterwards that the baby was perfectly healthy. And I loved the way Olga always told people that if she were meant to know the sex of the baby or know how it was going, God would have installed a window on her belly. Also, I read in one book that 94% of women could deliver naturally without any problem. So I decided to trust the process and be responsible for creating an environment where everything would live up to the vision I had created.

Finally Olga's visa was approved and we got married in a small ceremony in Oregon. We didn't have time to arrange a big ceremony as we were given 90 days to get married from the day she arrived, and we had no idea when the 90 days would start.

One night, when we were out shopping there just happened to be a farmers' market going on. Right outside the shop we were in was a woman advertising a home birth collective, run by a group of midwives. We got a lot of information that night and ended up contacting them later in the week to interview our potential midwives. Ellen and Kenna came over the next week and we talked through what we wanted to create in having our baby and what they could do for us. It really helped me more than anything to see that they had lots of experience and training and could handle the most common problems, should any occur. So Ellen would be our primary midwife and Kenna would be her backup. They would come by the house every other week to do checkups. Also, at that time Ellen was training Julie in midwifery, which would later prove to be a blessing.

For the next three and a half months we went through the basics of daily living. I worked, and Olga worked hard at being pregnant. And I mean this in the most positive way. Every day she took the time to walk a mile to the gym and swim for an hour in the pool. She took the time to eat really healthy food that would provide our child with a great source of natural nutrition. Olga took this time because she didn't want to take man-made, antenatal vitamins, which to her were not as good a source of nutrition as real healthy food could provide. She wanted our child to have only food that was from nature and full of life.

We took Bradley natural birth classes and this became one of my biggest learning experiences. We were in a class with five other couples who wanted to have their babies born naturally, but they were having hospital births. It was amazing for Olga and me to experience this class, where we spent half of each meeting learning how to defend ourselves from a hospital and their possible interventions when not needed or wanted. I remember in one class Olga was actually in tears hearing about all the problems with hospitals and we were not even going to one. It was an eye-opener to hear how they would tempt women to have some drugs regardless of what their wishes were. I was never more thankful for Olga's strength and determination to have our child at home in a loving environment.

Then came the big day. We were actually about two weeks from the projected due date, sitting in a cinema, watching *Star Wars I*. The big battle at the end was just starting when Olga got this very funny look on her face. I'm sure I would look like that too if my waters had just broken and my trousers were all wet. Well, needless to say, Olga never saw the end of the film and wouldn't do so for a couple more years. We headed home, just a couple of blocks away, and called the midwives...

[As we read next, Olga gave birth the next day in a birthing pool, supported by her midwives and husband. Back to Steve for the rest of the story...]

It was 3.40am in the morning, 29 hours from when Olga's waters first broke and Olga gave one more push and out came our beautiful baby girl right into my hands. We slowly brought her out of the water of the birthing pool and onto Olga's chest so mother and baby could start the bonding process.

It was great to have this time. No one carried her away, cleaned her up, probed or weighed her. We all just held each other and experienced the miracle we had just been given. I remember at one point about 13 minutes into working on the placenta Olga jumped and asked Ellen if she had long fingernails. She said, "No," and we went on. Then about a minute later Ellen was checking the progress of the placenta when she uttered those now famous words to us: "This is too hard for a placenta. Oh my god, you're having another baby!" And just as those words were leaving Ellen's lips Olga gave a push and out came another baby girl. Everyone in that room was completely amazed, and moved in quickly to deal with the extra child. For nine months no one knew there were two babies. I have to say the excitement in the room was pretty wonderful. Truly, we had a small miracle on our hands.

After some time, Olga delivered the placenta and we eventually brought the girls out of the birthing pool. Having Julie as an apprentice was again just perfect, as we needed three people to take the girls and the placenta out of the pool, while Ellen attended to Olga. We also had to remember which child came out first.

We had happened to wrap up the first girl in a yellow blanket and the second one in a blue one, so we created the rhyme 'blue two' which to this day still holds true. Olga had originally wanted to keep the placenta attached for 24 hours. This was to allow all the blood that is pushed into the placenta during the birth process to return to the child and also because of an old Russian spiritual tradition that recognises the placenta's importance in the development of the child. Well, with having just one placenta and two babies connected to it, this was not a good option. But we managed to go a couple of hours before I cut the cords. We then wrapped them up in blankets and brought Olga and the girls into the bedroom and put them in our bed for a well-deserved rest. Also, during this time the midwives took the time to get all the statistics like weight, height, and do all the other checks they do on newborn babies.

We spent the morning talking about the shock and beauty of what had just occurred, about the signs that had been there but that no one had picked up on, and for good reason. Ellen had, of course, never delivered twins at home and told us had she known that we were having them she would have sent us to a hospital. Knowing Olga like I do, I know she would have refused to go as she wanted the birth experience she had and really was fearful of what would have happened to her in the hospital.

We don't think hospitals are bad places, they are just not for us as we understand they have two goals: do the best they can to help women deliver babies, and make sure they avoid lawsuits. We had our girls 29 hours after the waters broke and if we had been in a hospital we would have had only 18 hours to deliver before they would have started to intervene and force the girls out. In reality, we had twins born perfectly, head first, with no complications. We didn't spend the nine months worrying about all that could go wrong, we focused on how it would go just right, and it did.

We didn't spend nine months worrying

A lot of people ask us how we could not have known we were having twins and all I can say is it was a series of events that helped us to create the birth experience we wanted. Throughout the birth Olga only gained 15 pounds and was actually six pounds lighter after the birth than the day she found out she was pregnant. So she had about 21 pounds total for the pregnancy and the girls weighed 4½ and 5 pounds. This was because she ate right, exercised and just took excellent care of herself—something most working women are not given the time to do these days. Also, Olga had really strong stomach muscles from many years of riding horses, which made the midwives' job of examining [palpating] her bump very difficult. The midwives didn't ever think to look for multiple heartbeats and, since we had chosen not to have a scan, the girls were able to support our goal by hiding from us all, so that they could be born at home in a beautiful, loving, peaceful and drug-free environment.

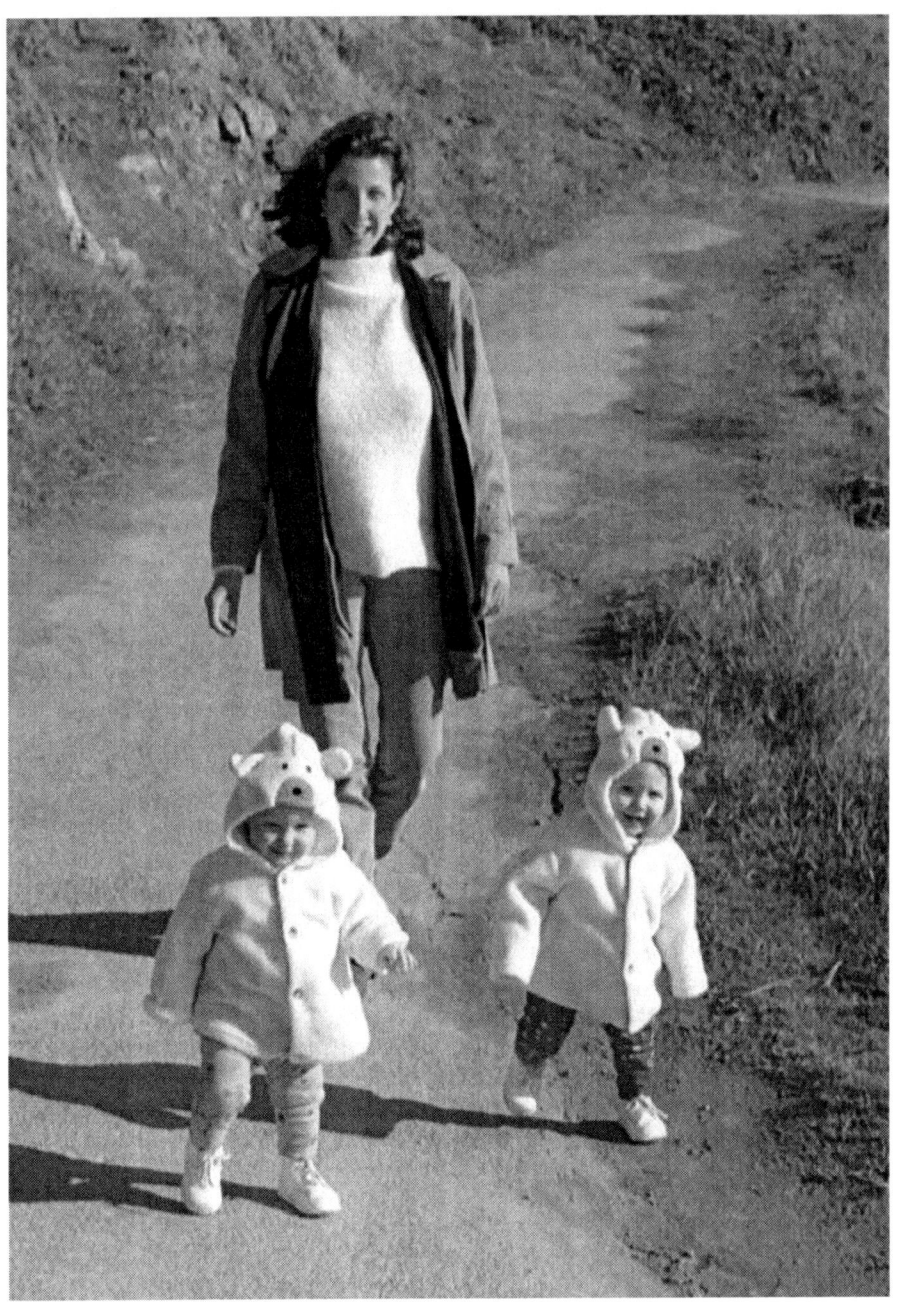

Olga with her two little girls

Olga's comments...

I had a beautiful and wonderful birth experience. I was very grateful for all the workshops I attended in Russia and for the Bradley classes in the USA. I was very conscious and confident about what I was doing. I think what helped me most on this journey was the deep belief that everything would be fine. I was taking care of my body—exercising and feeding it well—and it did a great job of getting through pregnancy and giving birth with all the wisdom of nature that it has inside it. In the classes in Moscow we discussed the process of birth through the experience of a child, which makes you understand that normal, healthy childbirth is the best way to bring a child into the world.

I am very grateful to Steven because he gave me a lot of love and support, which helped me to gain strength and confidence. During the birth we worked together like a great team. I am sure that creating a loving relationship in the family is very important for having a healthy, easy pregnancy and birth. It is not a rule but I believe that a happy woman with a positive attitude has a better chance to have an easy birth. Creating good relations depends on the people themselves.

In my opinion, these are the most important things, if you want to have a great, healthy birth:

♥ Have a deep knowledge of the benefits of healthy childbirth for both the child and the mother and make a conscious choice to do it 100% healthily. It is very important to select people (especially midwives or doctors) who will support and encourage you in your choices. It will never work when the woman says: "I will go to hospital and try to do it." There is a big chance that there will be a nurse who, after several hours of labour and pain, will say: "And now this is your last chance to get an epidural. Would you like it?" It's terribly hard to answer "No" when you're in pain.

♥ Have a deep belief in yourself that you can do it, trusting your own body with all its wisdom. Have a very positive attitude and a lot of gratitude for all the processes that are taking place within you.

♥ Take good care of your body. Have a very healthy, natural diet and do a lot of exercise (like swimming, walking, stretching).

♥ Consciously accept who you are and work to develop positive thoughts and a peaceful state of mind, and nurture a deep feeling of love for your child, yourself and the world. Work through the problems in your relationships with others (especially in your family) and within yourself.

Have a deep belief in yourself that you can do it!

Note from Sylvie:

In case you haven't already guessed, the photo on the cover is of Steve Mellor!

Having two or more...

Most of us only have one baby at a time, although increasingly couples are being taken by surprise as the multiple birth rate increases!

A pleasant surprise

Ulrike von Moltke

Daniel and his sister Dorothea were born naturally for the main reason, I believe, that we didn't know I would give birth to twins, so neither I nor the doctors would get nervous and I waited and moved about normally until the due date. It was in 1968 and scans were not routinely done yet. As I wasn't aware of any twins in my or Konrad's, my husband's, family—even though I was later reminded that my grandmother had also carried a twin inside her until it was discovered with some surgery after her firstborn baby!—I didn't suspect twins, even though I was enormous. But as my husband was very tall and my first son had weighed close to 9lb we all expected one big baby.

Labour started at 4.00am and when I got to the hospital they told me the baby would be born soon. But then it took hours, during which doctors and nurses and students listened endlessly to the babies' heartbeats, hearing one kind only faintly and never looking for a second kind. The doctor who was attending me at the time (in the USA) was famous for his 'spinals', but women often had problems with them afterwards, headaches etc, and anyway I preferred it all the natural way.

But finally, as by 11.00am nothing seemed to progress any more—I seem to remember that the baby was supposed to turn, which hadn't happened yet—the doctor decided to do a caesarean. When he told me I thought "Oh well, in that case I'm going to turn over to my side, which will ease the pain somewhat." As I had wanted to move things along I had all the time stayed on my back, the position that gave me the stronger labour pain. Anyway, very soon after I turned over, things began to move inside and I felt the urge to push. They could hardly get me to the birthing room and Dorothea was born with such urgency that I was sure all my lower parts had been ripped out along with her. Then I heard the doctor exclaim, "Oh, there's another one coming!" "Well I have to get on then," I said to myself, matter-of-factly. Nine minutes later Daniel was born quite easily, as his sister had prepared the way for him.

They each weighed close to 7lb, the girl a little over, the boy a little under. After being reassured that they were both all right I was greatly relieved. My husband and I were enormously happy and proud. I still see the other mother in my room receiving her baby for breastfeeding (no rooming-in yet back then) and I remember thinking, "The poor mother, she is only getting one baby." We felt so rich!

Absolute faith in my body

Kathryn Clarke

My twin daughters, Antonia and Charlotte, are now 13 months old. They are happy and healthy and absolutely wonderful. We decided to try for another baby when my first child, Marcus, was 7. When, at my 12-week scan, we found out it was twins I was absolutely petrified and my partner was delighted—he always had believed he was magic! The pregnancy went remarkably well, despite all the horror stories you hear and the various medical staff telling me to pack my bag at six months and finish work much earlier than I'd intended. The whole family were on tenterhooks for weeks. No one would go on holiday and, by eight months, people were starting to get very impatient. Personally, I was happy to wait as long as possible for the babies to arrive as—having experience of caring for one baby—I was well aware of the amount of work that would be involved.

Finally, six days before the due date, my waters broke at 3.00am. I jumped out of bed and got to the hospital as quickly as possible only to be told that I wasn't in labour and wouldn't be examined due to the risk of infection. I was given a bed on a ward and my partner was sent home.

Later that morning I had a visit from the consultant. She decided that she would give me until the following morning to go into labour naturally but that if I hadn't she felt it best to induce me. She then went on (to my absolute horror) to recommend an epidural. Her reason for this was that, as Twin 2 was breech, if there were any complications and I needed to have an emergency caesarean, I would be ready and wouldn't need to be knocked out. At this point I burst into tears and said that I really didn't want that. I was quite distressed to see how surprised all the staff seemed to be at this and when I later discussed it with a midwife she said that epidurals are now so commonplace that many mothers ask for them!

I'm not sure whether it was the shock of the consultant's visit or just the strength of my desire not to be induced but I very quickly began to experience a lot of pain and, on examination, was told that I was 6cm and really should be in the delivery suite.

I was so relieved that I was given total support in my decision to have no medical intervention when I met the midwife that was to deliver me. The only thing they insisted on was that a drip [a heparin lock] should be inserted into my hand in case I needed glucose. I was also given a gas and air 'contraption', which I didn't use—but I found the mouthpiece great for biting on!

After going into labour at about 12.30pm on 11 June, Charlotte Mary was born at 4.47pm (7lb) and Antonia Grace was born (bottom first and screaming) at 4.59pm (6lb 15oz).

I am so glad that I had the babies normally. I think that it is such an important experience and all part and parcel of becoming a mother. I was very scared of giving birth to twins and I must admit I have never experienced anything so painful but I found that the only way I could get through the pregnancy without being totally freaked out was to have absolute faith in my body. Throughout both the pregnancy and the birth I continued to remind myself that my body had done this before and therefore would be able to cope with it. Thankfully I was right and I do believe that, had I allowed them to give me an epidural, I would have felt I had cheated myself.

A rebirther's perspective

Gaia Pollini

It was really important to me to have a healthy birth because I'm a rebirther. Perhaps I should explain a bit about rebirthing. It's a breathing technique which opens a person up emotionally and energetically, i.e. physically.

Going through the process of rebirthing allowed me to access deep feelings and old memories, including that of my own birth experience. Rebirthers have actually discovered that the circumstances of a person's birth are mirrored in his or her life patterns. (For example, induced people feel often rushed or pushed into things and people who've had emergency caesareans give things up half way through.) This is why rebirthers feel that the way babies are born is so important and that a healthy birth is a good start to life—it simply results in less emotional baggage. People who are drawn to rebirthing are often aware of birth patterns repeating themselves in their adult life, or they are simply people who feel stuck and want to move on from old patterns and have heard that rebirthing works wonders in unblocking stuff, however old or deep it is (not just birth trauma). It is possible to heal almost anything with breathing and love. Rebirthing also makes you deeply aware of how fully aware a baby is before birth, as during sessions people often revisit antenatal states as well as birth and realise how much they were sensing and feeling and how much they knew about what was happening to their parents and around them.

I believe the positive attitude of my independent midwives also helped me because comments about 'twins always being early' can act like a negative mantra. In fact, our twins were born five days past their due date! I'm sure my midwives' positivity and faith were crucial. People are usually scared of being positive in case things go wrong. But there's really nothing to lose. If things go wrong, people can deal with it and then at least they haven't spent months worrying. It's best to stay positive and open and just have awareness of what's happening.

The only antenatal tests I had were two scans. I had the second one—another ordinary scan (i.e. not a nuchal one)—because I was bleeding, as I was the first time. However, the scan showed us everything was OK. A great deal of pressure was put on me to have more scans but I resisted this because my husband and I had decided we wouldn't have a termination anyway, even if it were recommended. In any case, the early scan had at least made us aware that the babies were non-identical (with two placentas and two sacs), which is useful information for a twin pregnancy.

I had a fantastic pregnancy. I was extremely open, which meant I wasn't always feeling great! However, I was very much in tune with myself, even in terms of what I ate. Although I'd been vegetarian before I got pregnant, when—a couple of months into the pregnancy—I really started fancying meat, I ate it whenever I wanted to. The love of being pregnant can help you be yourself even more strongly than before. I sensed my babies were loving the things they were experiencing through me.

I think babies are living beings the moment they are conceived and what you experience of the world, they also experience. I visualised myself giving birth at 40 weeks because I really wanted them to have plenty of time to grow. I also talked to them a lot, using any positive words I could think of. I also let myself feel excited and curious about the magical process of giving birth. I expected to have a fantastic pregnancy, so I did!

Overall, I'd say the most important thing for me was to stay away from other people's fears. I did not want to be near anybody being negative—which is why I didn't go to the hospital or near some of my friends. We just said, "We know what we're doing. We don't need your opinion." I hardly had any negative feelings myself. As far as comments about my due date went, every time anybody said, "When's your due date?" and I would tell them and they'd reply "Oh, they're going to be early because they're twins." I'd say "No! Mine are not!" And they weren't.

My labour lasted about 15 hours, then I had this amazing urge to start pushing. At that point I just wanted to give birth. My heart was set on giving my two babies a beautiful birth, so I made sure I stayed positive—even though I knew one of my babies was breech. (The midwives had been able to tell this just by palpating my bump. Fortunately, they also knew how to deliver breech babies.) Anyway, it went very smoothly—although I was exhausted afterwards! There was no tearing. I started breastfeeding straight away. It really couldn't have gone any better.

Then, when the twins were 8 months old, we bought a big camper van and drove to Italy. The idea was to look for our dream: a property and land where we could start a new life and business. We did find a beautiful house and land, and a year and a half later we moved to Italy permanently.

The twins are now 4 and I'm still breastfeeding them! (They have wanted a lot less milk since they turned 3, so it's only occasionally now.) I became vegan a year after the twins were born, and they were vegan too until they were 3. Then we all started eating other things—I'm far too relaxed to be too restrictive.

I just don't eat meat, and neither do my kids, only because by now we are not used to it any more. We now eat cheese, eggs and fish—with pulses every day (which the kids adore)—as well as seeds and a few nuts, soya, quinoa, etc.

If any other mother of twins—or singletons, for that matter—wants to breastfeed, I'd say stick with it, because it really does get easier and easier. The first few months are the hardest because the babies can't hold themselves up at all and with two it is harder, but it becomes second nature quite soon, both for Mum and the babies. One day you won't even remember what was so difficult. I had big problems in the first few days—it was so painful and I was so incredibly tired. Do contact a breastfeeding counsellor if you need to, even in the first week or two. Even if you have to pay, it's well worth the money. A breastfeeding counsellor will teach you positions and all the tricks, including breastfeeding lying down—which is a real lifesaver! It is actually easier to breastfeed twins, than prepare bottlefeeds for two. Remember, it does soon become easy.

After the initial problems, I loved it, and so did my kids. Within a week, all the pain was gone for me. I was just tired then! The advice and support I got at the beginning really helped make it a positive experience. And once it became positive and comfortable, there really was no reason to stop.

Before I sign off, I really want to add a bit about John, my husband. He was so, so important in the whole process. He was really positive and supportive and didn't get involved with the fear stuff. If we ever had different opinions, which was rare, he very openly talked about it and we always found solutions that felt right for both of us. He was respectful of my feelings and needs, without forgetting his own, which also needed to be worked through. We actually did the rebirthing sessions together and a couple of times the sessions ended up with me and the rebirther holding and cuddling and supporting him. Everybody's birth issues come up around birth, not just the mum's! It was so beautiful and free and loving that he could have his process and space around giving birth. It also allowed me to have more support when I needed it, particularly at the birth itself. At that time, he was just so, so amazing. He was there all the way, not just in body, but really with his whole self. We were truly together then just as we are now, as parents. I'm sure our children really feel this. We're in this together, the four of us.

I truly believe that whatever happens to anyone is just the perfect thing for them. Even if I had had a terrible birth, in the end it would have been OK. But, man, am I glad it went the way it did! Life is beautiful. If you're going through all this pregnancy thing now, I'd just say TRUST YOURSELF and allow yourself to feel all you need to feel. Allow yourself to be whatever you are. If you can, surround yourself with people who listen to you and who will support you in what you do. And listen to yourself at least as much as you listen to others, and possibly more. If other people's opinions clash with how you feel, don't dismiss yourself. You're important and special.

A pragmatic approach

Anon

I am a 40-year-old woman who gave birth to twins normally five months ago in an NHS hospital. It is possible! I did it with a lot of persistence and research, after several meetings with various midwives, consultants and hospital managers and by finding independent midwives and a consultant who supported me in trying for normal deliveries for our babies. With some luck, a very supportive partner and midwives, and a consultant who went beyond the call of duty by being available for me in the labour ward (though by my request, not in the delivery room) when he was not normally on call, I gave birth to the first twin in a birthing pool, and the second on land, without any drugs or intervention at 39 weeks and two days. Both babies were well and weighed in at just over and under 6lb. I would like to encourage other expectant twin mums or those with a high risk pregnancy to inform themselves of what the risks associated with their pregnancy are, what the birth options are with their various pros and cons and to persist in trying to lay the conditions and plans for a normal, healthy delivery, if that is what they want. Giving birth to our babies is one of the most satisfying, joyous and proud experiences I have had.

When you hear what some people have

Mave Denyer

I found out I was expecting triplets a few weeks before I went into labour. I was a bit shocked and I didn't quite believe it. This was back in the early 60s and I was having visits from the district nurse. She put on my card "Lots of limbs, go for an X-ray". That's how they discovered it. It wasn't as a result of infertility treatment and there was no family history of multiple births.

I already had two children. My son was then 3½ and my daughter was 20 months. I'd chosen to have them at home, as most people did 50 years ago. They'd both been very good experiences. As for the triplets' birth, obviously I would have liked to have had them at home too but when they discovered it would be triplets, they said it had to be hospital. There was no talk about having a caesarean, though. Nowadays, people seem to do caesareans at the drop of a hat. They are necessary at times, of course, but there was no need for one in my case.

It all started a week before Christmas, when I began having pangs, you know, contractions. They were born a bit early, as multiple births almost always are, but I can't remember how many weeks—about three, I think. Anyway, I went into hospital for about 24 hours or so and they said "Nothing's happening. Go home and come back again after your Christmas dinner." So I did.

I went back into hospital that night, when the waters broke. It was a case of "Call the ambulance immediately!" I'm not sure of the exact time but it was probably about 3 or 4 o'clock in the morning that I went in. And they were actually born just after 2 o'clock in the afternoon, about 12 hours later, the day after Christmas, within about 45 minutes of each other.

They were all born vaginally. I'm very happy that they were as normal as possible. No caesarean. No messing about. For both the babies' sake and for mine, too. There were no instruments or tearing or anything like that. No, I was lucky—when you hear of what some people have. Afterwards I felt as if I could push a bus over—I felt as if I could leap out of bed and do anything. But I didn't. There were no buses going by at the time. Yes, it was very exciting.

Now the triplets are almost 50. Jon's a bachelor with his own house and a Physics degree. His job involves the testing of many materials used in the building and construction industries. He plays badminton and meets his brothers and mates in a pub at least once a week. Tim now has three children—two boys and a girl—while Greg has three sons. They started their own gardening business a few years ago, with much help and support from their wives, and are now extremely busy. I often wonder if any of their customers think they are seeing double, which of course they are!

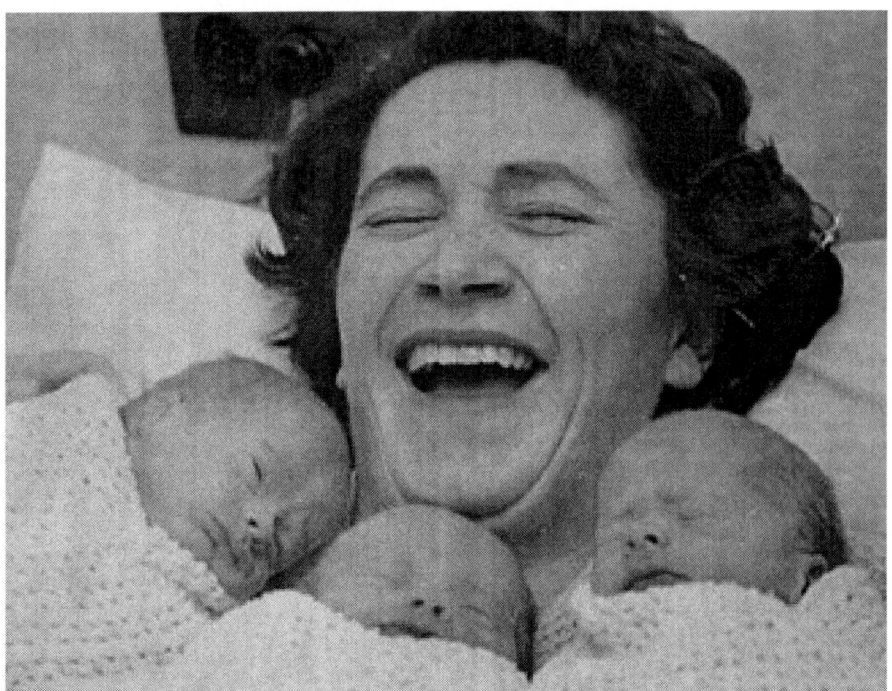

Mave with her newborn triplets

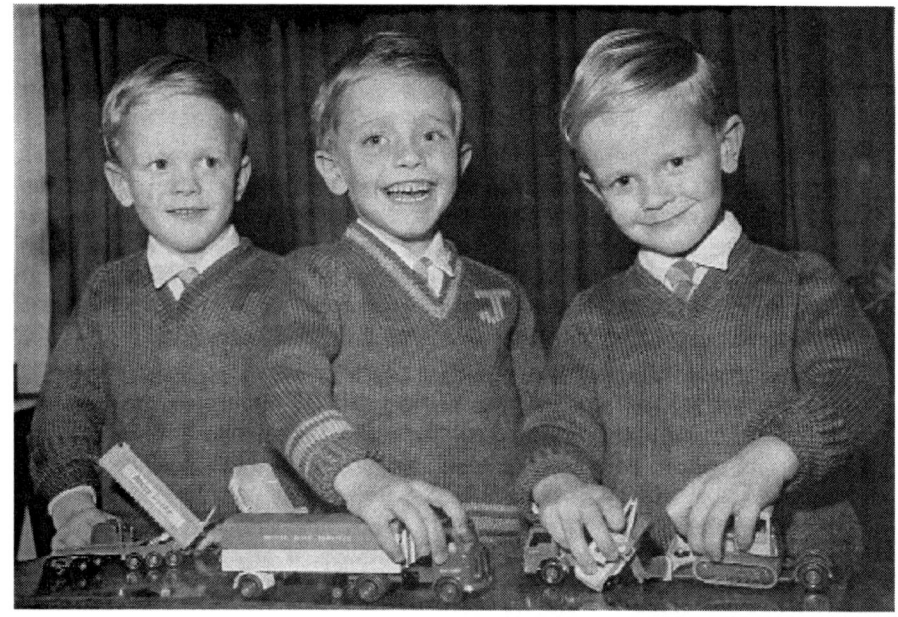

The three boys playing with their toys after school, aged 5

They were all born vaginally. I'm very happy they were.
No caesarean. No messing about.

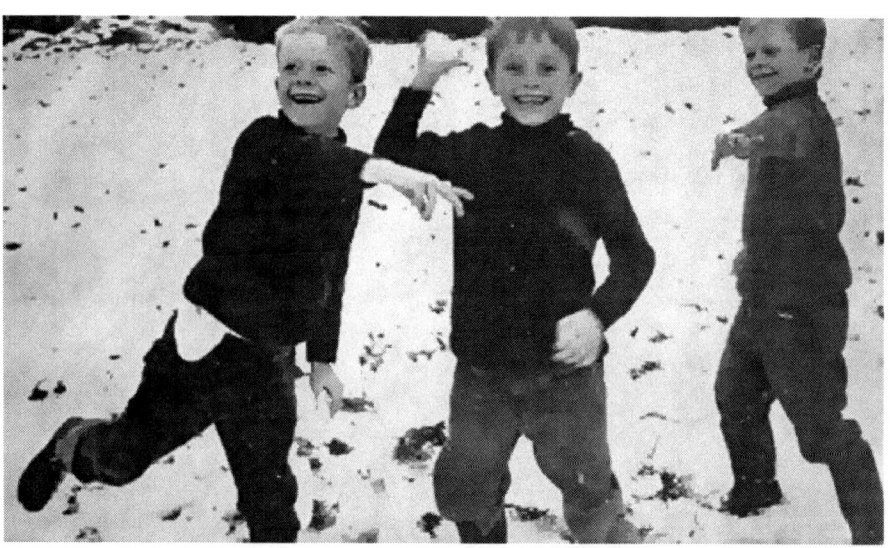

Having fun in the snow

Wellies to the rescue

Janet Hanton

In August 1999 in a small scanning room in a London hospital we were told some life-changing news. At 35 years old I was pregnant with my third child. Actually, third and fourth children as I had discovered at a previous scan that it was twins.

Since then, we had been away on holiday for three weeks, and had got used to the idea that things were not quite going as we had expected. We returned that day, just off the plane and very jet-lagged, for a further scan. My husband jokingly said "Just don't tell us there's another one!" We were stopped in our tracks by those unforgettable words: "Um... well, actually there is." I was pregnant with triplets. No IVF, no family history, we simply were that freak statistic—a spontaneous triplet pregnancy.

At 9.00pm on 30 November, the evening of my daughter's fifth birthday, my waters broke. I couldn't really believe it. I was only 28 weeks pregnant. Though tired during the pregnancy, things had gone well. I had been resting in bed for two hours each day, and had been feeling healthy and full of confidence. I had been told at the hospital: "As long as you get to 32 weeks, we're not too worried." I had been so sure that this pregnancy would go way beyond that date. I rationalised that I had already had two full-term pregnancies without any problems or complications. Clearly, my triplets would be born later rather than earlier. So confident was I that I used to pass over the 'premature baby' section in the books on multiple birth, sure that I wouldn't be needing that information.

We had taken on Caroline Flint to be our independent midwife as soon as I became pregnant with what we assumed to be our single third child. Caroline had been our midwife for our second child, and I had given birth to him at home. When planning to have a third child, I had thought that we would probably have another home birth. However, with the news that I was expecting triplets everything had to change.

Caroline tried, on our behalf, to find a consultant who was willing to consider a vaginal delivery of triplets. She did not have any success. Whilst we were not against the idea of having a caesarean if it were necessary for the babies' safety, we wanted my case considered on an individual basis. I had given birth two times before without any need for medical intervention and wanted someone to look at my particular case, consider all the options and make a safe and sensible judgement about the mode of delivery. The view seemed to be that triplets should always be born by planned caesarean and the fact that two of our babies were 'monochorionic' was given as a further reason for not having a vaginal delivery. (Incidentally, we have since discovered that all three babies are identical.) ['Monochorionic' means that two (or more) babies are developing in one chorion (bag), each in its own amniotic sac, inside the single chorion.]

One consultant, Donald Gibb, was prepared to consider a vaginal delivery, but his contract with my community hospital was to expire before my due date, and so he was unable to take my case on. We accepted that the babies would be born by caesarean.

When my waters broke, I immediately phoned Caroline, who said that she would come to the house and check me over. 15 minutes later I started to have contractions and so we arranged to meet at the hospital. The contractions were very quickly becoming regular and urgent-seeming. I felt panic-stricken, every minute seeming an eternity as we waited for my mother-in-law to arrive to look after our older two children.

We arrived at the check-in desk of the labour ward...
"I'm having contractions. I'm having triplets—I'm only 28 weeks."
"Take a seat. We don't have any rooms at the moment."
"But I think it's an emergency—I'm meant to be having a caesarean."
"We have other emergencies to deal with. Take a seat in Reception."

The situation seemed surreal. I was certain that I was in established labour and that things were happening at speed, and yet we couldn't seem to persuade the hospital staff to take us seriously. We went down to the reception area, which was out of sight of all staff. I felt quite despairing, pacing up and down, convinced that I would give birth to our babies right there.

Then, to our utter, utter relief, Caroline arrived, took one look at me and dived off down the corridor. She came rushing back, looking relieved. "Donald Gibb is here."

By a quirk of fate Donald Gibb was there on his second-to-last night at the hospital. Immediately, everything started to happen. We were rushed into a room as some poor woman was wheeled out into the corridor, and I have a hazy memory of Mr Gibb tearing the sheets off the bed. There were no intensive care cots available at the hospital and the plan was to transfer me by ambulance to another hospital, where there would be places for the babies once they were born. However, on examination I was already 9cm dilated (this only one hour after my waters had broken). It was then inevitable that the babies were to be delivered there and then.

I felt disbelief that this was happening to me. I was full of fear at what might happen to the babies, and indeed to me, and yet couldn't quite take the situation seriously. I found myself giggling inappropriately at Mr Gibb's wellington boots. The room filled up with people and equipment and I felt as though I was appearing in some bad hospital TV drama. At the same time, I was terrified. Instinctively, I turned my back on the room and knelt on all fours on the bed. This was the same position in which I had delivered my other two children and I couldn't imagine any other way. I remember Mr Gibb saying, "Do you want to deliver the first one like that?" and replying that I wanted to deliver them all like that. He said that he would see how things went.

The paediatric registrar kept appearing by my head to report on progress in the search for intensive care cots for the babies. It was mostly bad news. They couldn't find three intensive care cots available in one hospital, the babies might have to go to different hospitals, one might have to go to another town, etc... I became very agitated about this and remember Mr Gibb telling me not to worry, that it was their job, not ours, to sort this out, that our job was to get the babies out safely.

From that moment on, I felt a sense of calm. I felt that I had done everything I could. I was in expert hands and what now happened to the babies was out of my hands. I felt totally focused on giving birth. Although the room was full of people and I had a tube in my hand in case I needed a caesarean, I was able to block almost everything out. I had a scan during the labour, but it was so unobtrusive that I hardly noticed it. I knelt on the bed with my back to everyone and was aware only of Bruce (my husband) in front of me, Mr Gibb's voice, and Pam Wild (the other midwife) rubbing my back and reassuring me. I felt such faith in the people looking after me, and in my own ability to give birth that in spite of everything I felt calm and relaxed. I leant on Bruce, used gas and air and concentrated on counting my breaths, keeping them long and even. Exactly the same as I had done in giving birth to my other two children. I remember saying to Pam and Caroline "I'm pretending to have a home birth here."

At 10.30pm Kate was born. She was so tiny that it was not like the second stage of labour with my other children. It was more a question of trying to hardly push at all, to make her delivery really gentle. I didn't see or touch her, as she was taken straight to the resusitaire to be surrounded by a paediatric team and ventilated. I just had a chance for a quick look at her as she was wheeled past me on her way to SCBU [the Special Care Baby Unit], a scrap of humanity amidst a mass of tubes. I wasn't really able to focus on her birth as my mind and body both knew there were two more ahead. Then everything stopped. There were no contractions, and I lay against Bruce and felt as though I was almost asleep while we all waited. I had no sense of time at all, though in fact it was 40 minutes before Sophie was born. After 30 minutes Mr Gibb ruptured the membranes because she had some bradycardia [an abnormally slow or unsteady heart rhythm], and she was born shortly afterwards. 10 minutes after that, Louisa was born. All were born head down, and I was able to deliver all three kneeling on the bed with my back to the room. As with Kate, Sophie and Louisa were taken away immediately by their paediatric teams to be ventilated and we caught a brief look at them as they were wheeled away to SCBU. They weighed 2lb 9oz, 2lb 10oz and 2lb 11oz.

I asked for syntometrine, and shortly after the placenta had been delivered Bruce and I found ourselves alone in the room wondering whether it had all been a dream. We had no babies with us, all the medical staff had gone. It was only two and half hours since my waters had broken.

A little later Caroline and Pam took us down to SCBU to see the babies, where they were being held until transfer to another London hospital. We had been lucky as three intensive care cots had been found in one unit. I was in a wheelchair and felt as though I couldn't breathe properly. I couldn't really take it all in. The birth had left me feeling on a high, as though I could do anything. I felt fantastic, exhausted and confused. I couldn't relate emotionally to the three tiny bright red bodies in their incubators, covered with tubes, and hooked up to all kinds of machines. These didn't seem to be my babies. I was given a Polaroid picture of each one, and taken back to the ward. I didn't want to think about what had happened and asked for a sleeping tablet. That night Kate and Sophie were transferred and Louisa was transferred the next morning.

The babies spent the next two weeks in the neonatal intensive care unit. It was a very difficult and frightening time. The almost hourly ups and downs of each baby's progress meant an experience which could be likened to being on three roller coasters at once. And during this time we could do nothing but watch and wait. We couldn't hold them for many days and could do very little to help them. I was sustained during this time by the memory of their birth. The way in which I had given birth to them gave me a physical connection with them which I was not able to have during the first weeks of their lives. I also found it helpful that I was able to start expressing breastmilk for them. This was frozen until they were ready to begin breastfeeding.

After two weeks the babies were transferred back to the hospital where they were born. They spent a further five weeks in hospital before being discharged home at 36 weeks' gestation. I continued to express milk for them throughout their time in hospital and for some weeks once they came home. For 10 weeks they were exclusively fed with breastmilk, initially by tube and later from a bottle.

Kate, Sophie and Louisa are now happy, healthy 3½-year-olds.

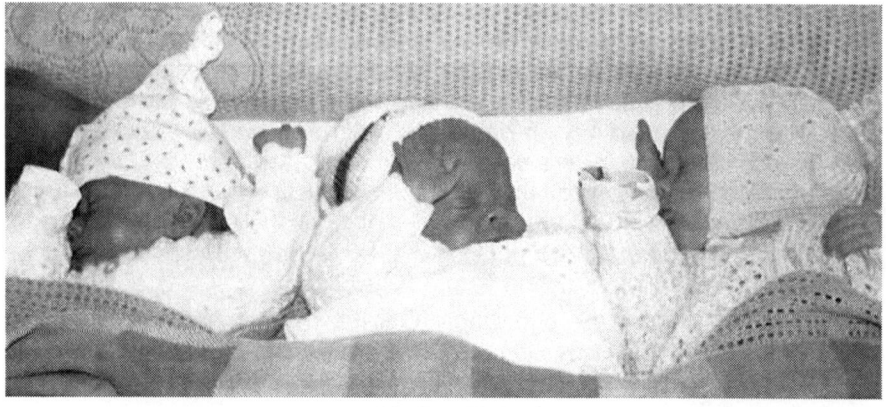

Kate, Sophie and Louisa (left to right) at 7 weeks old, just after they had come home

Coping with high risk and actual problems

As many as half, or even most, pregnant women will be considered 'high risk' at some point during their pregnancies. This isn't very surprising when you consider that many other everyday activities, such as crossing the road, are also pretty high risk. But what does risk assessment really mean and should it be cause for a great deal of concern?

If 'concern' means 'fear', then the answer should very definitely be "NO!" because we human beings produce a hormone called adrenaline when we're afraid (as you probably know) and it just so happens that this hormone is 'antagonistic' towards the main hormone of labour and birth, oxytocin. (In other words, when we produce adrenaline it's actually *impossible* for us to produce oxytocin, except in very unusual circumstances, such as the very moment of birth during an instinctual 'fetus ejection reflex'.) Since oxytocin is known as the 'hormone of love' amongst researchers (because of the types of behaviour that usually take place when a person is producing it), we need to focus on being loving, not fearful—while we are pregnant and we need to make sure the people around us are relaxed and loving too—not full of fear! This is simply, and worryingly, because any fear in another person near a pregnant woman will quickly be transferred to her...

Considering this hormonal backdrop to labour and birth and also the risk element of everyday life might help you to understand why the couples featured in this chapter chose to take the particular decisions they did. It might also help you to understand why the caregivers who attended these births did not intervene more dramatically and persistently, or more hastily.

A pregnancy problem

Justine Renwick

I gave birth to non-identical twin boys on 25 December 2001 in the John Radcliffe Hospital, Oxford—on Christmas Day. Here is a little background and the birth.

I already have one daughter, born in 1999 normally without pain relief or intervention until after the birth. I had a retained placenta so having done the 'hard bit' OK, I then had to have surgery to remove the placenta.

In September 2000 I had a missed miscarriage which resulted in surgery to remove 'products of conception'. Unfortunately, during the procedure the surgeon perforated my uterus!

I then conceived twins and was told, without any consideration for what I wanted, that I would have to have a caesarean section at 38 weeks. Once the hospital (not the John Radcliffe) checked my file and saw I had had a retained placenta and perforated uterus they said, well, that basically made it a definite section, no option. I was not happy with this and I asked to be referred to the John Radcliffe (JR) for a second opinion. The consultant at the JR—Lawrence Impey—was actually the consultant who had scanned me at 12 weeks and told me we were having twins; twins also happened to be his specialist area. He understood why I had been told a section at 38 weeks was necessary, due to the possible complications and strain my uterus would be under if I went into natural labour. However, he didn't rule out a normal, vaginal birth and said we would make that decision much nearer the time.

Pregnancy went well and I still didn't want a section. At 37 weeks the consultant agreed not to do a section at 38 weeks if the babies had not come naturally by then but he said he would not allow me to go beyond 39 weeks, so a section was booked for 39 weeks gestation. When asked if he thought I would get to 39 weeks, he said, "No, we'll see you next week, I reckon—about Christmas time." He was right!

On Christmas Eve itself I went into my local hospital to have baby movements monitored as all had gone a bit quiet. Everything was fine. On Christmas Eve whilst being monitored (at 5.00pm) I had the slightest Braxton Hicks, but nothing else. Came home and had supper and watched television. I had lower backache during the evening but no more than usual after a long day. Got into bed at 12.15am and at 12.30am had a show; called the hospital at 12.50am. We live about 45 miles from the JR! The midwife said to come in. Left home at 1.10am, got to the hospital at 1.50am; contractions were now four minutes apart but not severe or too painful. Alexander and Luc were born at 3.00am and 3.20am. They weighed 6lb 7oz and 6lb 5oz. Labour was basically two and a half hours.

The labour and birth... On arrival the midwife started monitoring me and I had one huge contraction. She said she would get the doctor to see if I was in labour properly but there probably was no hurry. I said I really thought this was it. The doctor came, had a look and gasped, saying, "9cm dilated!" and I'm saying, "Yes, and I want to push". The registrar came and said, "OK, we must get you into theatre to give us more room to manoeuvre and in case there's a problem." They wheeled me across to theatre. I had a drip in my arm to keep the contractions going once the first twin was born. I was then offered gas and air, which I used. A few hard pushes and Twin One (Alexander) was born—all healthy and already holding his head up on the table, where the paediatrician was checking him. Twin Two (Luc), who had been breech, turned and the second midwife sort of held my stomach so he could not turn back. I was then asked to do one really good push to push Luc into the birth canal, so he could not turn again. By this time the contractions had subsided and the midwife had to tell me I was having a contraction and to push. A few pushes and Luc was born—all healthy and also trying to hold his head up.

A few pushes and Luc was born—all healthy

Alex had come out with his hand along the side of his face, so I had torn and had to be stitched up. The placentas were slow to come but the midwife was fantastic, saying she had never been beaten yet by a placenta and out they plopped, actually fused together, so it looked like one.

And that was it. I had an Anti-D shot as I am Rhesus negative. The anaesthetic for the stitching was absolutely the worst and most painful bit of the whole procedure. By 5.30am or 6.00am I was on a ward.

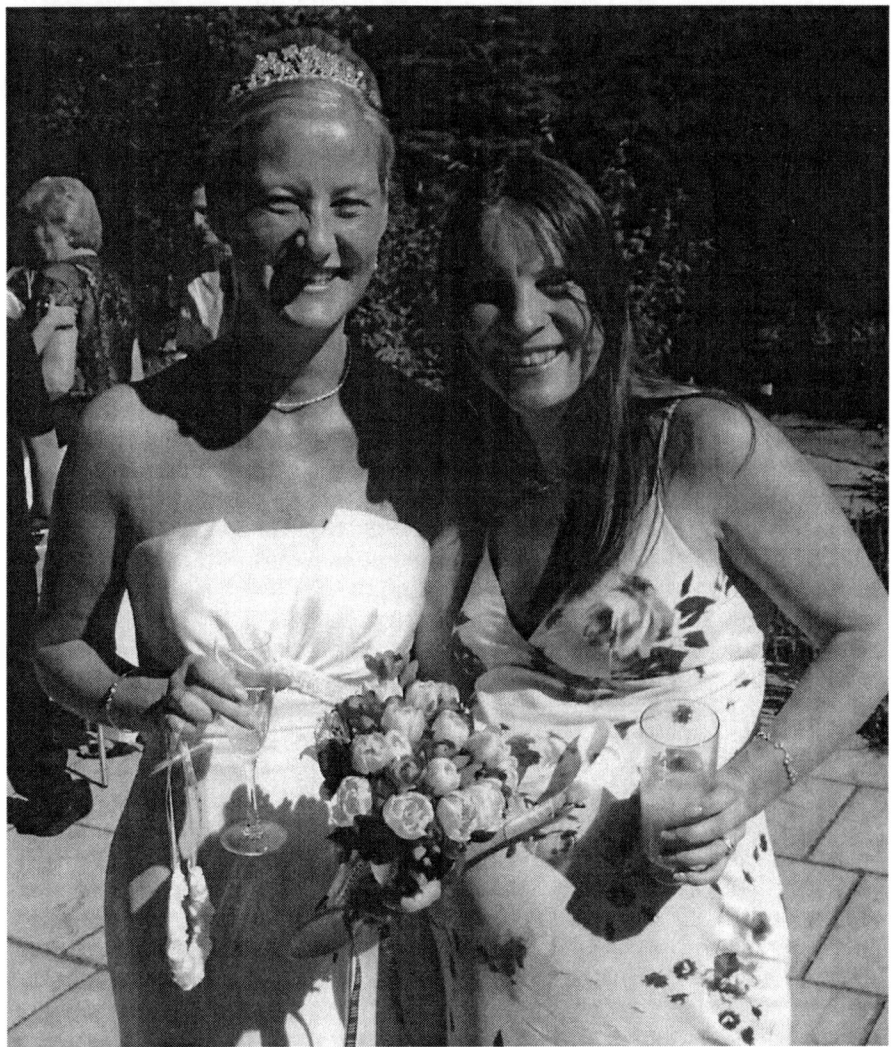

Sarah, an older mother (see overleaf), attending a wedding the day she went into labour!

Being 'elderly'

Sarah Cave

I gave birth the day after those wedding photos were taken. I'm 36 and Alice is my first baby—she's now 19 weeks old. I had a fabulous pregnancy. Loved all of it, even though I had slight morning sickness between Weeks 4 and 12. I was never actually sick—I just felt queasy and sensitive to smells. Amazingly, I also went off coffee and chocolate! Looking ahead to the birth, I decided I wanted to do without painkillers if I could because I felt it would be the best thing for the baby. And it was a fantastic birth. Not painless exactly, but really, really good.

My labour started when I walked in my front door, after I got back from that wedding! My waters seemed to be going. I felt wet and thought, "Surely that's not my waters breaking?" All night long I had contractions and I spent a lot of the time in bed, sort of asleep, but I kept on getting up for the contractions too. My husband wanted to keep me company and massage me, or whatever, but I just told him to go back to bed. "Just let me be. I just want to do this on my own," I told him.

We eventually went into the hospital at about 8.00 the next morning. When we got there, a midwife examined me. "I'll just go and get someone else to have a look at you," she said. "I'm not sure if my fingers are long enough." The second midwife said that, yes, I was definitely 10cm dilated. She asked me why we hadn't come in sooner. "I just wanted to be at home," I said, "just wanted to be quiet." They thought they'd better get me to the delivery room and suggested I get in a wheelchair. "Oh, I'll walk!" I said. Of course, I was naked by this time and one of the midwives tried to hold a towel or something round me, but I told them not to bother. I really couldn't care less who saw me by that stage! The midwife was fantastic—very calm. It was like having Mum at the birth. She looked after me and didn't let the doctors in. It was just me, my husband and the midwife. It was a really intimate and relaxed atmosphere. At one point, the midwife offered me gas and air but I thought, "No, I'll just keep going and see if I can manage," remembering it would be the best thing for the baby if I could. And of course, I did. Somehow, the time just went past.

No, I'll just keep going and see if I can manage... I did.

Alice is an 'angel baby'. She's feeding and sleeping well. She's very contented. The only blip was getting mastitis on four occasions from the second week after the birth until last week. I'd never heard of the condition until it happened. My biggest mistake was leaving the mastitis on the first occasion for over a week *before* going to the doctor's—and it was too late by then. So my advice to other new mums would be to get help any time you feel pain in the breast. Apart from that, I'd say enjoy every day! Don't give up on breastfeeding. I didn't and it's going great now. Alice has nearly doubled her birth weight and she's not even 6 months old yet! Good stuff, breastmilk.

Breaking family traditions

Michel Odent

One woman who contacted me belongs to a family that is familiar with caesarean birth. Her brother, her sister and herself were born by caesarean. When she gave birth for the first time, it was decided after a long trial of labour in hospital that the baby was too big for her and that she needed a caesarean: the baby was 9lb (4kg). While she was expecting her second baby she asked me if I would come to her home when the labour started because she wanted to try to give birth vaginally. My answer was: "Yes, if I'm not in Costa Rica".

The labour started during the night preceding my flight to Costa Rica. I could stay in her home until she was in advanced labour, so that when she arrived at the hospital with Liliana (her doula), she was not far from a point of no return. She eventually gave birth with the help of ventouse to another 9lb baby.

When she was expecting her third baby, she asked me again if I might come to her home when she was in labour. My answer was: "Yes, if I'm not in Italy".

The labour started two days before my flight to Italy. There were ideal conditions of privacy. I was following the progress of labour from another room, through the sound. Liliana who, as a doula, behaves like a cat, was around, evaluating the progress of labour with her own criteria—postures, sound, breathing patterns, etc. I did only one vaginal exam.

At 12 noon, the father left in order to make some arrangements so that the children could stay in the house of friends. Soon after, there was a series of powerful contractions—a real 'fetus ejection reflex'. At 12.45 the ecstatic mother gave birth to an 11lb (5kg) girl... no drugs, no tears, no episiotomy.

Unto the breech, dear baby

Esther Culpin

At a time when breech presentation is almost synonymous with caesarean section, I find it useful to write up the story of the easiest of my four deliveries. In this case, changing the birth environment absolutely transformed the way I gave birth. I set out to create a new birthing environment this time around as my previous births, although loosely defined as 'normal', were definitely not. The births of my three sons followed long and traumatic labours and I experienced excessive blood loss immediately afterwards. Overall, birth appeared to be extremely risky and to contemplate it all over again did not seem like a good idea. The solution to my difficult birth experiences could have been an elective caesarean section. Instead, I had the opportunity to look more closely at important issues that might have affected the way my first three births had turned out.

Giving birth at home was a really important factor for me because of the absolute freedom it gave me to do as I wished in labour. I needed to arrange for a midwife to be in attendance who would respect my need for a calm and undisturbed environment. Michel Odent was happy to assume this role and was noticeably unperturbed by my traumatic labour and delivery record!

When, after 30 weeks of pregnancy, my daughter was persistently a breech presentation, I made no change of plan. I was still happy, confident and looking forward to an easier birth in the privacy of my home. At this point technology could have taken over, but all the required information seemed to be available, literally through the midwife's hands. There was never a suggestion that I should undergo an external cephalic version (ECV) and, having experienced that procedure 14 years previously, I did not feel I wished to undergo it again. Although I was still aiming for the birth to be at home, I booked in at the maternity hospital just one mile away, in case admission to hospital and emergency treatment should be required. Local midwives, although acquainted with home birth, indicated their preference not to be involved with a breech birth if it was to be at home.

I went into labour a week after my due date. This time around, as part of a strategy for giving birth easily, I aimed to keep myself rested. This was achieved by not doing too many things in a day so that I would be able to cope with the rigours of labour whenever it started. As the process got underway, I found that being at home had a direct effect on the way I coped and on the optimism I felt. (Remember, the baby was breech, I had never experienced an easy birth before, and I was at home!)

On the domestic front I was assisted by my husband. Again, considering my history of traumas associated with giving birth, he was superb. His responsibilities were wide-ranging, but his priority was to maintain a safe, dark and secure environment for me, so that I should experience no disturbances. A birthing pool in the living room was filled with warm water, in case it should be needed for pain relief. The children went out to breakfast with their grandparents. For this birth, because I badly wanted things to progress easily, I did not wish to have any distractions at all.

For me, labour in any circumstances remains hard, but given that this time I would be able to adopt any position, and there were no outsiders coming in and out of the room (as there could easily be in the hospital setting), I felt that I was on the way to giving birth quickly and easily.

In fact, for the first time in my experience, labour progressed extremely quickly and I found myself trying to slow things down so that I would not give birth before assistance arrived! What was noticeable at this point was the lack of instructions I was given: Michel gathered silently all the information he needed to assess the situation. I was obviously ready to deliver and, because I was not directed in any way, I decided to get into the pool!

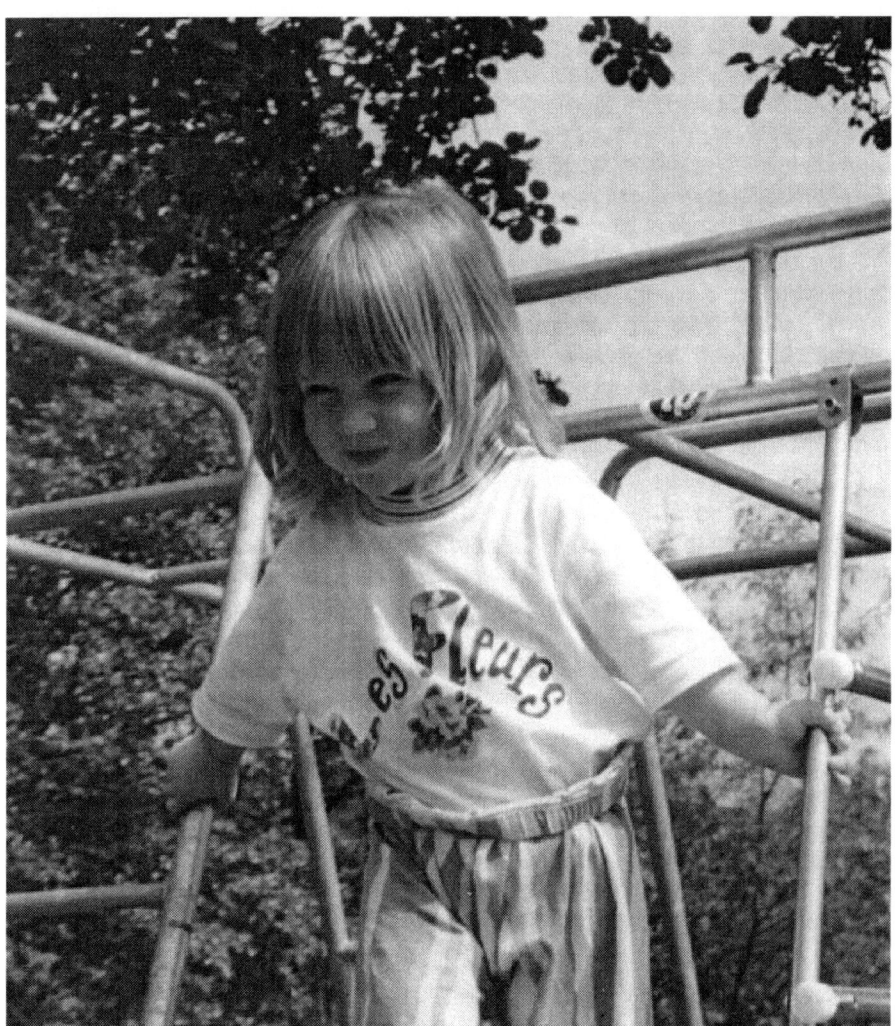

Little Ms Culpin having fun on the slide at the age of 2

At the next contraction and whilst standing upright, my baby's body was born. I was assisted out of the pool and supported from behind so I could maintain a standing position. Now there was a long pause while the cord, which was wrapped tightly three times around her neck, was unwound. Her head was deflected by inserting a finger into her mouth before her head was delivered. During these few critical minutes there was no discussion about whether I had a girl or a boy.

My daughter lay on the carpet, motionless at first. But, in that situation, I was her life support, just as I had been all along. The fact that I was personally and actively involved in those early moments was of prime importance to me, whatever the outcome would be. I trusted deeply that my daughter would live and I felt that my participation in every way would give her an optimal chance. But, whatever, we were together in this and that's how it should be, whatever the outcome.

The position that I adopted at this point, immediately after her birth, was also extremely advantageous. I was leaning over my daughter, who was lying on the ground. This was the optimal position in the early moments of her life: it aided the natural compression of the uterus and meant that the baby could be readily gathered up as soon as this became appropriate. There was no cutting of the cord, no touching of my abdomen and no administration of artificial hormones.

After a little while, I moved on to a nearby sofa and instinctively lay on my side with the baby. The move from floor to sofa was easily undertaken, the cord remaining slack in the process. I was now in that wonderful time following birth but had not experienced any preceding trauma.

Probably within the hour, the placenta separated and by that time the cord was lifeless and could be cut and tied. I really preferred the idea that the cord would not be cut in the early moments following birth since this would maximise all the benefits to the baby. Blood loss was minimal. I had experienced a totally physiological third stage.

This birth turned out to be easy and untraumatic. Very simple measures were taken to change the factors surrounding birth and these appeared to make a huge difference: I was at home, I had freedom to move around as I wished, I was not watched by anybody (including my husband) and I had faith in the 'midwife' [Michel Odent]. From my perspective as the mother, the fact that my baby was in a breech position proved to be a secondary consideration.

Speedy, timely intervention at birth

Nuala OSullivan

I booked Michel Odent for my second daughter's birth, having complete confidence in him and his approach to birth. I had first met Michel when I was being a birthing partner for a friend and watched her beautiful daughter emerging like a lithe Excalibur from the depths of the birthing pool. Michel had then helped me to deliver Ciara, respecting my labouring foibles. He not only accepted that I would soak anyone who came near me but also reassured the local beat police that in fact a child was being born and no one was being murdered, despite the scary screams! His gentle consistency and faith in the labouring mother inspired confidence and allowed me to deliver as I had not believed I could.

Ciara had been 17 days late so when my due date of New Year's Eve came and went and all the women in my yoga class delivered before me, I wasn't unusually perturbed. On 14 January I made the journey to nursery, with my toddler dancing forwards and back to keep pace with my slow gait. I was expecting that the 17 hours of Ciara's birth would be divided by three for this baby. Contractions were steady but only 10 minutes apart so I still felt safe and anyway knew people in the shops and houses all the way to the nursery. Her key worker and other parents were all excited for me and still maintained their enthusiasm when a day later we had only progressed to five minutes apart as we made the journey even more slowly. On Friday afternoon we went for a walk with the children and I sat on a see-saw with another parent to try to encourage contractions along. By the evening labour had become established.

I bathed Ciara, walking around our tiny bathroom as she sang to me. Once she was asleep I called Michel, who came to see me, reminding me to call at any time.

My dear friend, Fee, arrived and sat with me. With night and our relaxed energy there seemed to be a lull and, although they never stopped, the contractions didn't seem as powerful as they had been. All night we sat up awake but contractions weren't developing. We looked at the birthing space with the empty birthing pool dominating my bedroom. Located over a cement archway the bedroom was deemed the best room for taking the weight of a filled pool. I had scented oils, the same ones I'd used for Ciara and candles at the ready—remembering how light sensitive I'd been the last time and how I'd craved the cocoon of my room. The freezer had frozen lemon ice cubes for sipping later and there was plenty of cooled water in the fridge.

I was getting worried by the slow development of contractions but by 6am on Saturday contractions had re-established themselves more earnestly. Sally arrived early on Saturday followed by Danuta, my homeopath, and Jill Furmanovsky who had taken such precious pictures of Ciara's birth. Michel dropped in on his way for a swim, untroubled by what felt like established labour to me. I felt partially put out that my 'serious' labour didn't warrant any further attention and partially reassured that he was off for a swim, so delivery wasn't imminent.

Between contractions I dressed Ciara and she went off for the day with friends. The day passed in a blur. I liked the sounds of the women around me as they talked, prepared meals and got on with other things somewhere on the periphery of my consciousness. I did not engage well with the group by this stage, didn't want people near me. All my social senses dulled, my need for attention became muted. Jill came and gave me a massage at the base of my spine as I had been rocking and could not get comfortable. It was welcome and comforting, and her gentle energy was calming. Mostly, I felt the need to be alone—to have them all somewhere near me but as background, rather than with me.

Michel seemed to materialise as stages progressed and then to fade into the background again. Fee came and sat quietly in the room, when she wasn't making drinks for everyone. Sally cared for Ciara and timed contractions from the kitchen, attuned to my sounds. Danuta checked on me and monitored changes in mood and energy but only sporadically as Michel was keen for me to be left in peace. He instructed that no one should make eye contact with me or disturb me unnecessarily. His protection of the birthing room was useful to me as I took myself out to deal with the contractions. I became acutely sensitive not only to light but even to whispering sounds from the other room.

Nothing was expected of anyone, so each found their own role.

I felt sick. The waves of nausea were welcome as they meant that my body was starting to work and would bring my baby to me. Contractions escalated and I was aware of how tired I had become after two sleepless nights so I began using self-hypnosis. As the contraction began I took myself out and when it released I came back in again. I begged to go into the pool and was heartened when I saw them filling it. It paced me through the next few contractions and gave me something new to focus on.

The light faded and Ciara arrived home. Sally bathed her and I kept going in and out to change her story tape over—I was driven by an odd duty to be there for Ciara, even while labouring.

Because of Ciara, I think, there was no screaming this time and the contractions waned when I shifted attention from them to her. Ciara's birth had been loudly vociferous. As a trained soprano I had released each contraction with treble notes, as round and powerful as the labour itself. My neighbours knew I was labouring and were unconcerned but a passing beat pair called in to ensure that no murderous assault was in progress. Michel had protected me from prying eyes and the presence of extraneous visitors. Although the police wanted to see me, to set their fears to rest, Michel reassured them that all was as it should be and that I was having a baby. They returned the next day to ascertain that a baby really had been born with the police officer declaring that the sound had been 'bloodcurdling' and the woman police officer resolved never to have a baby after what she had heard! Yet Ciara's birth had been beautiful to me.

Sally lay down with Ciara and I could hear her telling Ciara about the night she was born, answering Ciara's questions, until they both drifted off to sleep.

The landscape of pain established...
I kept telling myself I could do 'just that much'

The landscape of pain established. If I had been told two hours or four hours more it would have helped me to put a shape and sense to it but there was no way of predicting. I was 5cm and in the pool.

Contractions took me out and when they abated I floated. I kept telling myself I could do 'just that much' again. I drank and sipped ice cubes but couldn't communicate with anyone. I was glad they were there somewhere nearby, but not near me. I tried counting, moving, dancing, going in and out of the water until I was too tired to move from the warm water.

I was glad people were nearby, but not near me

Michel came and monitored me and told me the baby was fine and coping well. That was all I needed to hear. I could keep going if the baby was coping, so this time I stood still to allow monitoring and didn't drench anyone. I could feel my leg wriggling ready to move away. I found the enforced sedentary pose intrusive but I brought all my reasoning to bear on keeping still for long enough for him to take a good reading. Then he moved away again, quietly leaving me to my own space, the journey of my baby and me, unfettered.

Contractions kept challenging me. Just as I got used to one level a new one opened up, demanding my full concentration. Sounds became excruciatingly magnified as all my senses heightened. I shouted to them in the kitchen to be quiet even though my own sounds were louder and they had only been whispering. Still, all complied with the unreasonable request.

My waters exploded like a water bomb in the pool. Sudden, shocking. Danuta was topping up the pool and took the opportunity to ask me how I felt... I told her: "Everything irritates me". "Nox Vomica," she muttered, and went off to find a remedy. I heard the book pages flipping from the kitchen as she studied. It was all too noisy. The pages were like flapping sails to my ears.

Within an hour of taking the remedy I went from 5cm to 10cm dilation and delivered. The last hour I found exhausting. The baby was aligned along my spine [a posterior labour] and not my front as Ciara had been. The pool no longer comforted me and I wanted to get out. I felt hot, cold and unable to find the centre of the contraction any more. My drive towards the birth and meeting my new baby wavered and I felt emotional and hesitant for the first time in over nine months. My 43-week pregnancy was drawing to a close. From nowhere I started to panic. I believed that I would not be able to bring my baby into the world. Then I felt the baby wasn't capable of going on this arduous journey.

Even as I crossed the bridge of transition I knew that if I could only get through it I would be able to deliver successfully.

Pushing started then and confidence returned. Here was a part I understood. I had a role and something to do with each contraction. I felt myself organising my body's responses and planning how I would greet the new contraction. I got out of the pool thinking that I needed to open my bowels and that once I had I could have my baby. Once in the bathroom I realised that the sensation was confused because my baby was on the base of my spine and was in fact crowning.

I called out to them: "She's crowning!" As I staggered back to the bedroom, I noted to myself that even I had started to adopt Ciara's 'little sister' notions. The different voices passing on what I'd said didn't irritate me this time

Michel materialised, allowing me to find my position and my own connection with the contraction. I leant my hands against the wall and pushed. A head emerged with the cord round its neck and an arm up beside it, making the top centile head even wider. Michel deftly slipped the cord over the head. Another contraction and the rest of the baby slithered out, caught by Michel as I collapsed in a heap.

Tired out but terrified. Because there was no sound. No crying.

A little grey daughter with no muscle tone and no sound.

3.6kg, 59cm and inert.

Michel was cradling my baby and sucking out her nose and throat. I splashed water from the pool to baptise her, desperate to do something for her. Then I heard the indignant sound of Isolda's own voice. Michel rewarded me by handing me my wailing daughter. Perfect.

Sally took her while the placenta was delivered. Despite having size 4 feet (related to the pelvis size?) and an 8lb (3.6kg) baby I didn't need any stitches! Everyone came around me to admire and meet Isolda Lily, each loving face welcome to me now. I bathed with her and then Ciara woke to meet her 'little sister'.

Ciara is 17 and taking 'A' levels now, and hoping to study to become a midwife in September. Isolda is 14 and 5' 6", preparing for GCSEs and aiming to be either CEO of ICI or a catwalk model—whichever happens first! In the meantime, she is curiously delighted with how she has turned out... which is refreshing for a teenager.

A long, long labour

Elaine Batchelor

I was a midwife before I had any children and my first baby, Sophie, was born at home after 16 hours of normal but painful labour—there had been 24 hours of pre-labour, which I didn't count. I had the help of a supportive husband and a fab midwife.

> Being a second baby, I thought she would tumble out after three hours of manageable labour but I was wrong

Amy Rose is my middle daughter and she is 13 years old now. Being a second baby I thought that Amy would, of course, tumble out of me after three hours of manageable labour, but I was wrong.

I was three days past my due date and on my way to see the osteopath for treatment for lower back pain. I had a very strong contraction and then another, five minutes later, but that was all. On the osteopath's table the baby was writhing about like a bag of puppies and the poor chap was a bit taken aback at the sight of it. I didn't mention the contractions I had had as this may have made him even more nervous about treating me.

I had a show and contractions started straight away

I got home and prepared tea as usual and then Peter came home at 7.00pm as usual. At around 9 o'clock I had a show and contractions started every 5 minutes straight away—similar to my first labour. I had no idea what position my baby was in and it was before the days when I was so keen on optimal fetal positioning so I hadn't bothered to ask. By 11.00pm the contractions were very painful and every four minutes (I thought I must be at least 8cm by now). Oh, how exciting—the baby would be born soon!

I woke Peter and said "Peter, labour has started." He said, "Have the waters broken?" I said, "No." He said, "Wake me when they do." At around midnight I was fed up on my own and I could not lie down so I made him get up and keep me company. We decided to call the midwife who came round and got things ready, etc and as there was no sign of the baby by 1.00am I agreed to being examined. Oh joy... I was 2cm dilated. We plodded on through the night as I could not sleep. The midwife went away (she only lived round the corner) and Peter went back to bed. At around 8.00am we all met up again, plus Sophie, aged 3½, and Grandma, aged 70—someone who was going to look after Sophie. I also tried to call a friend who was going to come and care for all of us as our doula, but her telephone was out of order.

During the day I ate, but vomited everything back. I walked and swayed and knelt and was on all fours and used the shower, which was horrible by the way. At around lunch time I was pronounced 5cm dilated. My midwife suggested she break the waters to speed things up and as I was exhausted I agreed. As it was, it was so hard to do that she never knew whether they went or not and no fluid actually came out at all—very odd! Because I had been so sure of my super quick and easy labour I had not thought it necessary to hire a TENS machine, or pool, or anything at all to help me in labour.

Not much happened for a while after the waters were broken. Sophie and Grandma went off to the nursery Christmas party and came back with various little glittery things they had made. They were quite sad not to find any babies at home, just mummy slogging it out with contractions every five minutes still.

My midwife carried on supporting me with her quiet confidence, knowing it would be fine

The GP called in. I didn't want to see him so requested he be kept outside the door. (You can do things like that in your own home.) Of course, this labour was going on much longer than usual for a second baby and in hospital they would have been pressurising me to have an oxytocin drip to speed it all up but my midwife was from the days when all births were at home unless it was life or death and she carried on supporting me with her quiet confidence, knowing that it would be fine.

At one point at around 3.00pm I was in such agony that I secretly thought of going to hospital for an epidural. But I was pronounced 8cm dilated, which made it all seem much better. Sophie came and went as she wished and was not at all disturbed by seeing or hearing me in labour, as opposed to Grandma who was finding it all quite hard going. Sophie came along and put a tiny elastoplast on my tummy to see if it would help. She also drew lots of pictures, lying on the bedroom floor.

At 6.00pm I was fully dilated and had started pushing spontaneously. 30 minutes later, just after Sophie had popped up onto the bed next to me, out came Amy Rose. The second stage was a doddle! Things I had not prepared Sophie for were that Amy was covered in vernix, which Sophie found most odd, and that the baby had no clothes on, at which she was very surprised. She also spent quite a bit of time calling her baby Jesus as she was born at Christmas and Sophie had just been to a Nativity that day.

After Amy was born I had more agony in the form of raging afterpains. I was in agony all over again! I was having a physiological third stage so should have been encouraged to change position and to push a bit with each afterpain but I wasn't, so it was taking a while. Again, I didn't have the knowledge then that I have now. The GP came along to check the baby over and was anxious to see the placenta out before he went off to a Christmas party in Surrey. (I didn't know he had his wife waiting outside in the car as well.) He stepped in and started pushing and pulling on various bits of me and my cord until I could not bear it any more so I shouted at him to "get off me and don't touch me again" and I pulled his hand off my abdomen. He backed off and the midwife encouraged me to push and the placenta came out just fine. In the end I think he prolonged the third stage with his impatience. After that he went away and everything settled down again. I had a bath and we all had tea and it was all fine.

Why did it take so long? Because my baby was in a posterior position and I didn't know. Things were very different for the birth of No.3! I had optimal fetal positioning, the pool, the doula and very direct instructions from everyone about what to do in third stage. [Optimal fetal positioning is basically about making sure you don't lean back and relax while you're pregnant—at any time! While you're in bed you need to lie on your left side, not on your back. Leaning forward helps the baby get into an anterior position, which means a shorter and less painful labour.] I had also changed to a new GP as I didn't want a repeat of the brutal treatment I had had with Amy's third stage.

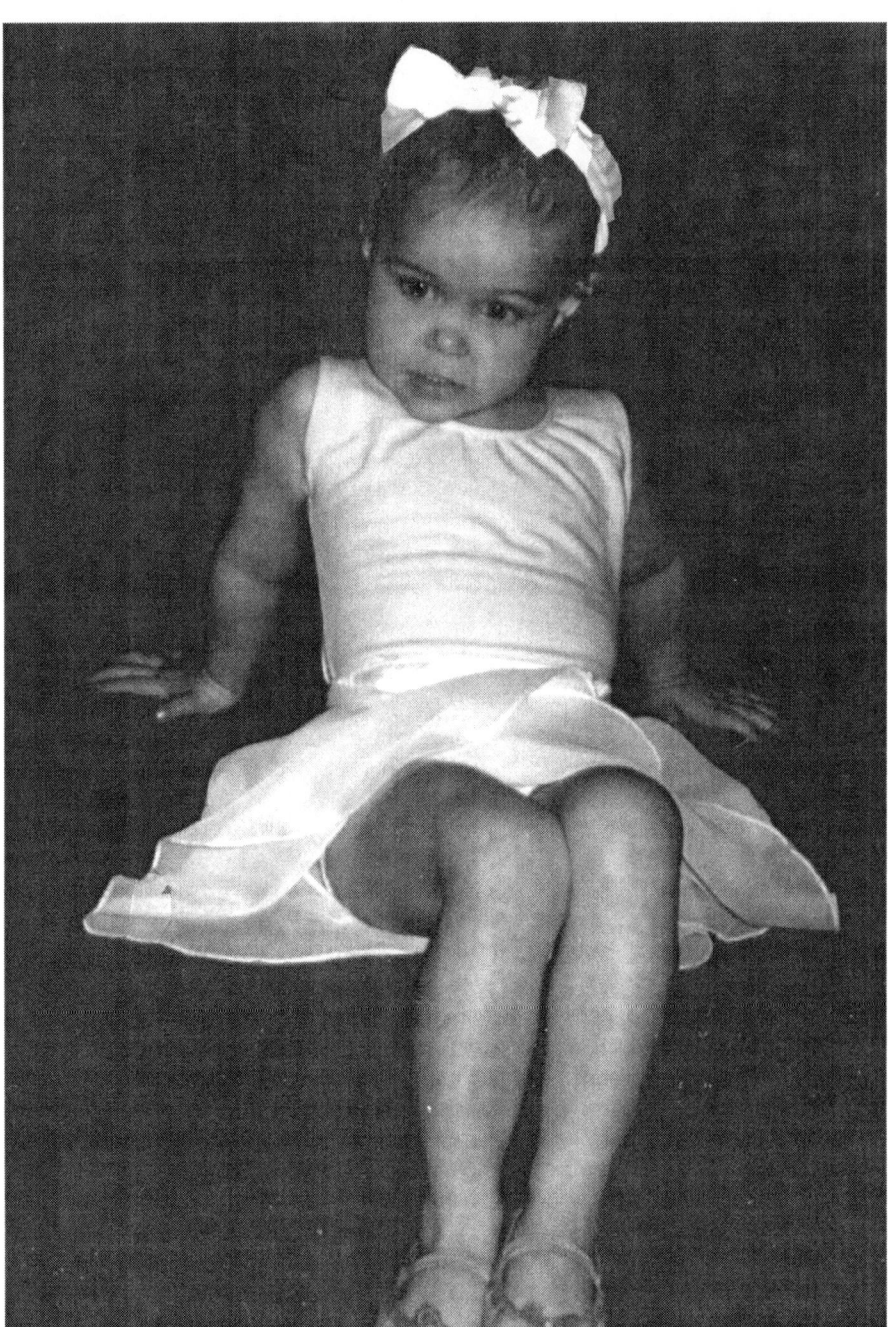

Here's Isolda, Nuala's 'baby' (aged 3), taking a moment to reflect before a ballet class (Remember Nuala's account on pages 72-76?)

Sophie was shocked that the midwife was clearly not going to take the baby away with her at any of her postnatal visits, but at age 16 years she has learned to live with it (just).

Questions none of us feel able to answer are: When did my labour start? Whatever happened to my membranes and the presumed fluid round my baby? There was never any sign of it before, during or after the birth! In hospital the presumption would have been that they went the day before (and that I had not noticed all that fluid pouring out of my vagina as I went about my business) and that my baby and I would need antibiotics (probably intravenous) to stop us dying of an overwhelming infection. But we were fine.

All in all, thank goodness I was at home with a midwife who had the confidence to see an unusual but normal labour. It saved us from a lot of medical intervention which could have had an adverse effect on the condition of me and my baby.

Unexplained bleeding

Anon

Zack (my first baby)

Zack's birth was as peaceful as a hospital birth can be. I was apparently not eligible for a home birth because of bleeding during the pregnancy. I had been given steroid injections to mature his lungs but fortunately the bleeding had stopped and I was home for most of the pregnancy. I was a few days shy of my due date when the real contractions started. I returned to my mother's house, had a meal and waited to be ready to go to the hospital. A few hours later we called and told them my pains were a few minutes apart but my waters hadn't broken. We headed in and were met by a midwife who stuck me on the monitor and was very careful to explain that things could take a long time as this was my first baby but that I would do just fine.

As soon as I got my own room I was given a mattress on the floor, a birthing ball and some cushions, and was encouraged to move around as much as possible, breathe through my pains and ask if I wanted any pain relief. (I had written in my birth plan that I wanted to be able to move around.) We were left to ourselves for as long as we wanted, I was provided with plenty of water to drink and food was available, but I didn't want any. By the time my husband arrived I was ready for some pain relief. The midwife suggested I get into the big bath (not a birthing pool). I did, but quickly became uncomfortable. For some reason being in the water made me feel a bit claustrophobic and edgy. I chose to have gas and air, which was provided quickly by the midwife, who also listened to the baby's heartbeat at that time, before leaving us alone again afterwards.

The only time the midwife came in the room was when I wanted her for something. She would then ask if she could listen in to the heartbeat with the Sonicaid, but she only did that if I was OK with it. (Sometimes I didn't want her near my tummy.) [A Sonicaid is a device for listening to the baby's heartbeat, which uses ultrasound. The Pinard, does not use ultrasound so is preferred by some mothers. However, the Sonicaid does have the advantage that it can be used very unobtrusively and some models also work underwater.] I was only examined vaginally when I felt like pushing. My waters still hadn't broken so the midwife asked me if I wanted her to break them or leave them alone. I decided to get the waters broken because I was feeling very tired as it was nearly midnight. The bag of waters was broken quickly and without causing me discomfort so it wasn't as bad as I had expected. We established that it was definitely time to push—I did need telling with my first. I wasn't sure I was ready! I had been very confident that I would get through the labour and her attitude really helped. If I became discouraged at any point she was great at getting me to focus and concentrate on the end goal of having my baby. Once he was born she helped me latch him straight onto my breast as I had requested in my birth plan, which she had clearly read because she did everything I had asked.

Once the placenta had been born I went for a quick wash while Simon and Mum dressed the baby. The midwife left us alone again and told us that she would write up her notes outside so we could have some peace and quiet.

So, the birth was really exactly as I wanted it. I was active and left alone by the midwife as much as possible. She kept her voice low and spoke to me directly rather than to my mum or husband. I don't think that anything could have been better, given that it was not a home birth.

Jamie (my fourth baby)

Jamie was born at 33 weeks. I had been admitted to the hospital 10 days before his birth with bleeding. I was given daily ultrasound scans because every time I went on the monitor his heartbeat was dipping down very low. I spent most of every day lying on my left side. I was allowed to head home for an hour or two here and there to see my other children.

The consultant had said that he thought my bleeding was coming from my placenta and probably had been in all my pregnancies—but eventually decided it must have been caused by micro-abruptions. Previous doctors had not been so sure and had simply described it as 'unexplained'. The plan had been to leave me on bed rest until 37 weeks and then to induce labour. The only thing that was complicating this plan was the dips in my baby's heartbeat. I was told that if they started to last any longer I would be rushed off for a C-section. I had also been given steroid injections again to mature the baby's lungs.

The contractions didn't show on the monitor

I had been having some contractions for the whole time I had been in the hospital but nothing that really showed up on the monitors. I was pleasantly surprised to find that the doctors and midwives looking after me were prepared to actually feel my bump and look and see that the contractions were real!

At just 33 weeks I woke up in the morning to more pains. I stood up to go to the bathroom and I felt a gush of water. I had never had my waters break spontaneously before so headed off to the toilet to see if I had wet myself, I was so unsure! Once I was sure my waters had broken I called my husband and told him to come in. There was nothing to be done to slow my labour because of the bleeding I was getting. The midwife and doctor were very calm and collected and examined me to see how fast things were going. I was already at 3-4 cm so we moved down to the labour ward. This was the first time it was just my husband and me at the birth. My mum was at our house with the other children.

Once I was settled into the right room things went pretty fast. I was ready to push after an hour or so. Unfortunately, the paediatricians were very impatient to get into the room as I was still pushing. The door to my room was open and although the midwife drew a curtain across I was very aware that there were several people standing around waiting for me to give birth!

I asked loudly for everyone to "GET OUT!" and the midwife went and told them to leave and close the door behind them and that she would tell them when the baby arrived.

I was so nervous when I was pushing because I was not sure what to expect from such an early baby. The doctors had been to see me and told me some of what we could possibly expect but really nothing can prepare you for going into labour early like that.

The midwife was great for keeping me focused but the baby's heartbeat was dipping very low for long periods so she had to tell me to push as hard as I could to get him out fast. I had wanted to do it in my own time again but I don't think there was much choice. He was pretty small so was easier to push out than my other babies.

He cried when he was born and was very active. He was put onto my chest for a minute or so. After that he was taken away to Special Care to be assessed. I decided to have the injection to speed my placenta up so I could get to him as soon as possible. I was desperate to go and see him but as soon as the placenta was born I passed some huge blood clots so I was advised to wait a while. A nurse came with a photo for me to see and at that point I persuaded them to let me go and see him, using a wheelchair!

Jamie was in Special Care for 11 days. I held him after two days and breastfed him after three. I was home two days after the birth because there was nowhere for me to stay. The Special Care Unit was not geared up for a parent to stay with the baby, which is a huge shame.

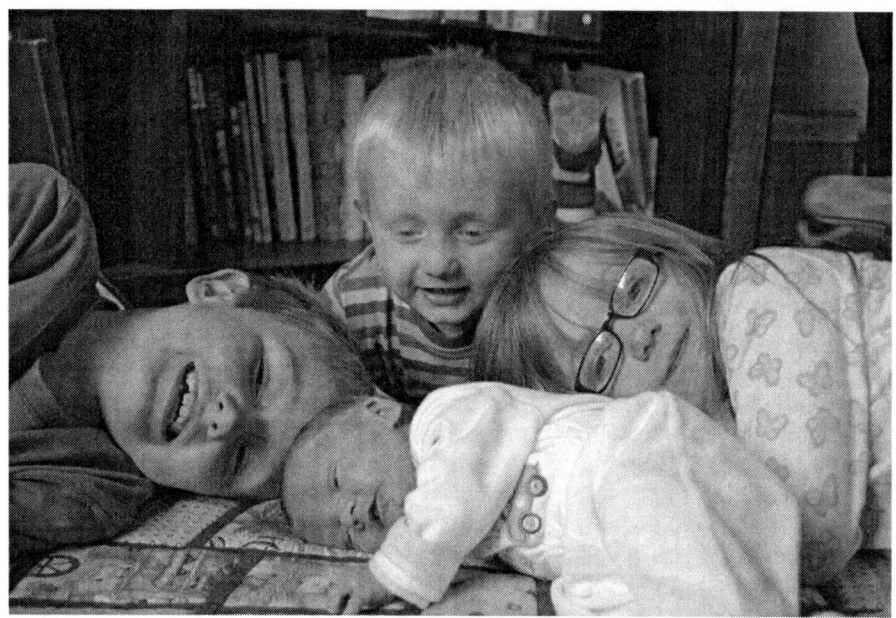

The four children who were born after this unexplained bleeding

Understandable, dangerous bleeding

Anon

Having had one fairly straightforward birth, it came as a shock when I realised things can go wrong in pregnancy. My second pregnancy was ectopic so at nine weeks I had emergency surgery. Luckily, I did not lose the fallopian tubes but they did end up damaged. So, in order to have any future children the only option was to go through a lengthy, costly IVF programme. We were extremely lucky to be successful on the first attempt, where I became pregnant with twins. However, fairly early on I developed hyper-stimulation (painful swelling) and one of the twins died by the 10-week scan. (A lot of early scans are performed with IVF to detect ectopic pregnancies and check that everything is developing normally.)

> I was told to expect some minor bleeding. They said bleeding can be a response to all the vaginal scans.

As I had lost one of the babies I was told to expect some minor bleeding. They also mentioned that bleeding can be a response to all the vaginal scans... So when I had some small bleeds before the 13-week scan I was not surprised, but a little worried.

At the 13-week scan I was told I had placenta praevia, which was fairly low down, but was told that for most women by the mid-term scan and certainly by 28 weeks the placenta moves sideways and away from the cervix, along with the growth of the baby. I continued to get small bleeds and was up and down to the hospital like a yoyo. At the mid-term scan (20 weeks) I was told that I had major placenta praevia, being classed as Grade 4+ (1 being minor and 4+ being serious). This meant that the placenta would not be able to move away from the cervix as it was completely covering the os, and in some places was adhered to the cervix. I was told I would not be able to give birth normally and would have to have a caesarean.

At 25 weeks I started to have a fairly heavy bleed and was admitted for the duration of my pregnancy. Luckily, I stopped bleeding but had to keep a cannula in [a device for a drip] just in case I started to haemorrhage. I was allowed home occasionally as long as someone was with me 24 hours a day and I was within 10 minutes of the hospital. This is because I would have to be on the operating table within 20 minutes if I started to haemorrhage, as the worst-case scenario is death of both mother and child. At my 28-week scan the earlier diagnosis was confirmed—there was no way I was getting away with a normal birth.

I started to have contractions at 32 weeks, which caused problems as I was not allowed to go into labour. (This is because the cervix dilates in labour and this would mean the placenta would rip, causing a major haemorrhage.) After being monitored on the labour ward to see the strength and frequency of contractions I had an emergency caesarean under general anaesthetic.

[It was necessary to have a general anaesthetic in this case for the sake of speed. An epidural takes much longer to set up and sometimes doesn't become effective the first time it is administered—which then means needing to try again.]

I was extremely poorly after the caesarean because I did end up having a haemorrhage, as well as some sort of reaction to the anaesthetic. My daughter spent a short time on the special baby ward before being whisked into the Neonatal Unit as she was having breathing difficulties. Mother and baby are now both fine—and the 'baby' is now 3 years old!

In general, I would definitely be on the pro 'normal birth' side of things, wherever possible. My pregnancy was clinical and from the outset not only was it a traumatic experience, I was unable to hold my baby for nearly two weeks after she was born. I was not aware I had had a baby until four hours after the birth.

Caesareans as a birth option are ridiculous. Mothers 'opting' to have an elective caesarean when it is not a necessity are totally nuts! I did not recover properly until four months after the birth. It is major abdominal surgery.

Giving birth too early

Krisanne Collard

In July 1994, my husband and I moved to the little town of Canon City, Colorado. We had no family in the state—in fact, we had no family within a day's drive. I found out I was pregnant within two weeks of the move. We were ecstatic! We had tried to get pregnant for three years and suffered a miscarriage eight months before. We were finally going to have the baby we had dreamt about for so long.

I had my first antenatal appointment at the end of September when I was 11 weeks pregnant. The doctor asked me to provide a urine sample, confirmed I was pregnant and told me my due date would be 4 March. He sent the rest of my sample off, so the lab could run all of the standard tests for new mums. He told me everything looked wonderful and I would be able to hear the heartbeat at my next appointment. I scheduled my next appointment for a month later and my husband and I left the office overjoyed at the thought everything was fine. We went to Wal-Mart and looked at all of the pretty baby things, dreaming of what our new baby's room would look like.

The doctor called me three days after the appointment and asked to see me in his office later that day. He sat us both down and gave us the bad news. All of the standard tests he had run indicated that I no longer had a viable pregnancy. Our baby was probably no longer alive. He scheduled a scan for Monday, just to be 'sure'. It was then Friday. All weekend we worried and panicked. By Monday, I had convinced myself that she was indeed dead—that we would have to try again. When I lay down on the table and told the technician why I was there, she had tears in her eyes as she prepared to take a look. For two agonising minutes, all was quiet. Then, she screamed "Oh my God! Look! Your baby's moving!" Sure enough, there was my little fighter, angry at the world—wriggling and trying to get comfortable. Her heartbeat was strong. My doctor never had an explanation for the incorrect test results.

For the next two months, my pregnancy went by the book. I had some morning sickness and started to get a bump. I felt her move for the first time on my birthday (14 November). We bought baby stuff and started to decorate the baby's room. We were the happiest parents in the world!

But, on 30 November, 24 weeks into my pregnancy, everything went black. I woke up with a dull ache in my lower back. I didn't think much of it till I started bleeding at about noon. I called my doctor and my husband, who rushed me to the local hospital. I was immediately hooked up to a fetal monitor and checked for dilation. I was already 5cm and her feet were in the birth canal. She was coming breech. Next thing I knew, I was being prepped for an immediate C-section. I was sobbing, screaming and confused. No one had time to talk to me—no one would let me know how the baby was doing. My husband and I were terrified!

When I woke up, I was in the recovery room. All I can remember was asking for a drink of water. I didn't ask about my baby because I thought she was dead. I just started crying—mourning her already. After about half an hour, another nurse came into the room. I asked her, "Was it a boy or a girl?" She smiled at me and said, "You have a beautiful little girl!" I was confused. She hadn't spoken in the past tense and she was happy. My daughter was still alive!

I was moved into a private room and my doctor came to talk to me. He told me that my daughter had been born weighing only 1lb 12oz and only 13½ inches long. He said she came out kicking and screaming, angry at the world, but she was VERY sick. They were transporting her to a level three NICU (Neonatal Intensive Care Unit) at Memorial Hospital, an hour away, in Colorado Springs. He told me that there was only a 30% chance that she was going to make it through the night. I didn't get to see her before they took her away. As I recovered from the C-section, I called the hospital she was in three times a day to check on her. She had been put on a special oscillating ventilator, I was told, and required maximum oxygen doses to keep her saturation up. They said she had got an infection from me and was very sick. I had a bladder infection I didn't know about (I have always been symptom-less) and she had come early because she was too sick to stay in my womb. They assured me over and over that she was a fighter and was going to be fine. They encouraged me to talk to her over the phone—but I felt silly because I hadn't even met her yet. Since we now felt she was going to make it, we decided on a name—Kaia Michele— a strong Norwegian name for a very brave little girl.

When I was released from my local hospital, four days after her birth, my husband and I immediately went to visit Kaia. When I walked into the NICU, nothing could have prepared me for what I saw. She was the size of two Barbie dolls stuck together. She had the blue bilirubin lights on her and tubes and wires everywhere. Her skin was translucent and her veins showed through her skin. I looked around, hoping to see 'my' baby in another bed. I looked back at Kaia. The nurse urged me closer and turned off the blue lights so I could take a closer look. I was terrified. The nurse urged me to touch her and talk to her—let her know I was there. I hesitated. She looked like she would break if I touched her. I started to talk to her but it took 15 minutes to finally get up the nerve to touch her. When I did, her alarms went off. I jerked my hand back as the nurse came over. She had to rub her till her heart started again. I couldn't handle it— my baby had rejected me—I left the nursery in tears and went home.

The next night, as we were eating dinner, I burst into tears. My husband took my hand and led me to the sofa. He put my shoes on and said, "Let's go— Mummy needs a baby fix." We drove the hour to Memorial Hospital. All the way there, I told my husband that THIS time I was going to be strong. I was going to count her toes and talk to her and let her know how loved she was. I was so excited!

However, when I got to her side and touched her, her alarms sounded again. The nurse had to start her heart yet again. I just sat there for the next 30 minutes and looked at her, crying. Why didn't my baby love me, I wondered? A nurse specialist named Theresa Kledzik (nicknamed 'The Whisper Lady') came over to talk to me. She asked me if I had held my baby yet. I just laughed and said that Kaia couldn't tolerate me touching her—I would kill her if I tried to hold her. Theresa just smiled at me and asked me to follow her into the other room. She gave me a gown, told me to take off my bra and shirt and put the gown on with the opening in the front. I was in shock as I changed.

When I walked back into the nursery, there were three nurses getting Kaia ready to be transferred to my chest. It took about 15 minutes for them to get her ready and I got more and more nervous every second. I changed my mind about 10 times, but the nurses didn't pay me any attention. I sat down in a strange-looking chair. (I learnt later that it was specially designed to be used with babies on oscillating ventilators.) They laid Kaia on my chest, on her tummy, skin-to-skin with me. Her head was resting above my heart and her tiny feet were curled up in my hand. The tubes and wires were taped to my gown. I stared at the monitors as she wriggled into a comfortable position. I knew they were going to sound. I held my breath. She calmed down after about five minutes and stopped moving. I thought she was dead. I tried to make sense of the monitors. I called Theresa over and asked if I had killed her. She just laughed and said, "No, she's happy!" I looked down at Kaia and noticed the peaceful look on her face. I looked back up at Theresa and smiled. My daughter had just made me feel like a Mum for the very first time!

I was able to hold Kaia every day for two hours. I couldn't get to the hospital fast enough every day to share that special time with her. Within a few days, I was able to transfer her to my chest all by myself, even with the tubes and wires everywhere. I was always disappointed when our time together came to an end. She responded very well to it and her oxygen requirements lowered during every session. She never had any episodes where she stopped breathing (apnoeas) or periods where her heart stopped (bradyas) while I held her. She would just go into a deep, healing sleep and actually tolerated my touch when she was on the warming table. The future was looking very promising for her.

When she was two weeks old, she had trouble getting comfortable on my chest. I wound up putting her back after only half an hour. I spent another hour with her, then headed home. When I got there, there was a message on my answering machine telling me to immediately return to the hospital. My husband and I rushed back just in time to say goodbye as they rushed her into theatre. They had no idea what was wrong and no idea how long we would have to wait. Four hours later, the Neonatal Surgeon came out and told us she was going to be fine. She had had a small perforation at the end of her large intestines and the surgeon had done a colostomy.

We got to see her within an hour. She had a huge bandage on her tummy and they had given her paralysing drugs. She looked so little and sick. I cried as I held her hand for the next two hours. The nurses assured me I'd be able to hold her again in a few days. I missed her so much.

I visited her the next morning. She was very uncomfortable and was requiring maximum pain medication doses. She wriggled and cried (silently because of the ventilator tube in her mouth). Finally, after an hour of seeing her suffer, the nurse said "Hold your baby, she needs you!" I leapt at the chance and got her out of bed myself—making sure not to put too much pressure on her tummy. The nurse came over a few minutes later to check on us. She smiled. Kaia was actually lying on her newly operated-on tummy, sleeping peacefully. I held her for the full two hours and she didn't even need her next dose of pain medicine! I was on top of the world. I had got to hold and comfort my child!

Kaia required another operation, at 3 weeks old, to modify her colostomy. She was moved to the Intermediate Nursery after two months, and came home on oxygen and a heart monitor a month later, on 27 February, two weeks before her due date.

She went back into the NICU two weeks later for an eye operation to correct ROP (retinopathy of prematurity), which is common in premature babies who have been on oxygen for long periods of time.

A month after that—she was 4½ months old by this time—she had a fundoplication [an operation in which the top of the stomach is wrapped around the oesophagus, creating a valve] to correct severe reflux. We had to feed her through a tube (called a G-tube) for the next four months.

When she was 8½ months old, she had her final operation to reconnect her colostomy and take out the feeding tube. She remained on oxygen and a heart monitor continuously till she was a year old. This meant lugging around a 15lb oxygen tank and a 10lb heart monitor everywhere. People were very curious. In the grocery and department stores I was given strange looks or stopped and asked 100 questions before I could continue my shopping. We didn't get out much because it was such a hassle.

That first year of Kaia's life was the most stressful year of my own life. There were so many things to do: doctor's appointments, operations, therapy sessions, medications and colostomy bag changes. And so many milestones: first smiles, first words, first steps, first hugs! I was on a roller coaster that didn't seem to have an end in sight. I joined a local playgroup and an online premature baby support group when Kaia was 6 months old. Both groups gave me so much love and support. They kept me from going insane. There are MANY premature baby support groups on the Internet and probably one in your own area. To find the one that's right for you join several—don't limit yourself to just one. Every support group is different and unique. Your hospital will be able to tell you if there's a local support group near you.

At our NICU reunion party in August 1995 Kaia was 9 months old. I ran into the nurse specialist who had encouraged me to hold my daughter the first time, Theresa Kledzik. We talked for almost an hour about 'kangaroo care'. That's what she called the skin-to-skin contact I had had with Kaia. I asked her if all babies were able to be kangarooed and she told me that I had been very lucky. Most parents in other hospitals weren't able to kangaroo their babies as soon as I was. Most parents had to wait till their babies were 'stable', off the ventilator or three pounds before they were allowed to hold them. I was shocked! Kaia would have been over two months old if I had had to wait. I couldn't imagine having to wait that long to feel like a mum.

When I got home, I immediately told my online support group about what I had learnt. Most wrote back asking what kangaroo care was and how they could do it. They had never heard of it before. I searched the Internet and found only one site that even mentioned kangaroo care. I was upset. How many other babies had to suffer without the loving touch of their parents? I emailed Theresa and she sent me all of the literature and research she had on the subject.

There was so much, it took days to go through it all. I was amazed at all I learnt and angry that more hospitals didn't embrace kangaroo care. Here is just a glimpse of the amazing discoveries I made...

♥ Kangaroo care—originally called 'kangaroo mother care'—was developed in Bogotá, Colombia in July 1977 by neonatologists Edgar Rey and Hector Martinez. It received worldwide publicity in 1983 when the startling success of the approach became known. The mortality rate for premature babies in Bogotá had been 70% (39% in the US at that time) due to lack of power and reliable equipment (such as ventilators and incubators). After getting mums to carry their babies continuously in slings on their chests, the mortality rate decreased to 30%!

♥ Research has shown that mums and babies have a natural thermal synchrony. When Mum thinks her baby is getting too cool, her body heats up in response. When Mum thinks her baby is too hot, she cools down. Sorry, Dad, this only seems to happen with mums.

♥ The skin-to-skin contact helps in milk production and milk letdown. It is very important for mothers of premature babies to pump and store their milk for the time when the baby can start eating. The breastmilk of a mother who has given birth prematurely is tolerated by the baby's immature digestive system more easily than formula.

♥ Apnoea (interruptions in normal breathing), bradycardia (severe heart rate decreases) and tachycardia (severe heart rate increases) decrease or disappear altogether because kangaroo care regulates breathing and stabilises heart rates. These episodes are VERY common in premature babies and can easily lead to death or lack of oxygen to the brain, which could cause brain damage.

- ♥ Kangaroo care stimulates the baby to gain weight more rapidly and be discharged up to 50% sooner because there are greater periods of deep sleep that enable the premature baby's body to heal faster.
- ♥ Kangaroo care can also be done with full-term babies who have colic. Colic is believed by many to be a baby's inability to transition from one sleep-state to another. Kangaroo care allows babies to enter into the deepest sleep state with ease. Most preemies that are kangarooed never suffer with colic. Mine didn't.
- ♥ Premature babies who are kangarooed during treatments (such as 'heel sticks' to check the amount of oxygen in the blood—an hourly requirement for premature babies on a ventilator) experience far less discomfort and require no extra pain medication during these painful procedures. Kaia didn't even seem to notice the treatments if she was being kangarooed.

After telling my online support group about what I had learnt, I was encouraged to set up a website to educate the world about the wonders of kangaroo care. One of my online friends helped me design the website www.geocities.com/roopage and several mums wrote stories about their first kangaroo care experience. I received so many wonderful stories, I decided to compile them all into a tiny booklet that I could send to NICUs and parents across the world. *Kangarooing Our Little Miracles* lets parents, nurses and doctors share the emotional joy kangaroo care brings to babies and parents. Most parents shared with me that by writing down their emotions, it helped with their healing process. I gave away over 200 booklets within the first year and received at least 15 emails a month from parents, neonatologists and nurses who wanted to implement kangaroo care in their hospitals. It feels wonderful to be an instigator.

In October 1996, I was asked to speak at the First International Congress of Kangaroo Care in Baltimore, MD. I was both flattered and nervous. I blew the minds of several nurses and neonatologists in the audience when I told them about my kangaroo care experience. They couldn't believe that I had been able to hold her on a ventilator (an oscillating one at that), or hold her when she was so unstable. They actually gasped when I told them about her reaction to being kangarooed after tummy surgery. They all cheered at the end of my speech when I told them that all babies deserve to feel their mother's and father's love and all parents deserve the opportunity to be parents, not visitors.

My 'preemie' (premature baby) is now 8 years old and going into 3rd grade. Where has the time gone? She is doing wonderfully at school and has no lasting effects of being born prematurely. She is sweet and kind and funny. She puts a smile on my face every day. The other day, when we were swimming at the local pool, another child asked her why her tummy was all messed up. (She insisted on getting a bikini even though her massive scars showed.) I held my breath, wondering if I should step in and help her explain. My eyes filled with tears as she said, proudly, "I was born the size of two Barbie dolls. I have these scars to show me how strong I had to be to live." I know that I helped give her that strength. I am so proud of her and thankful to Memorial Hospital of Colorado Springs for giving me the opportunity to be her mum!

We found out I was pregnant again in December 1995. My pregnancy was uncomplicated. My doctor checked me every two weeks for bladder infections. (I was treated for two during my pregnancy.) My doctor informed me that the antenatal pills I took with Kaia might have played a role in her early birth because they contained a high content of iodine, which I am highly allergic to. He switched me to an antenatal vitamin that contained no iodine. With Kaia, whenever I had missed one pill, I spotted. After missing two, I had Kaia. I am still very allergic to iodine and have to watch which multivitamins I take and keep salt out of my diet as much as possible. Even though I showed no signs of premature labour (i.e. contractions or bleeding), my doctor put me on terbulatine (used to stop contractions) at 28 weeks to be sure I wouldn't go into premature labour. I strongly encourage women who have ANY problems with their pregnancy to talk to their consultant. Don't just let it go. Even a small problem could snowball and mean life or death for your baby.

My mum teased me as I went through the summer months uncomfortable and VERY pregnant. Every time I would complain about how miserable I was, she would laugh and say, "YOU are the one who wants to see what it's like to carry a baby to term. You are going the full 40, young lady!"

My doctor left for his first holiday ever on 1 August, a Friday, right after my 36-week appointment. He took me off the terbulatine and told me that I was NOT going to have her till he got back! I just laughed and told him that I wanted to have her that weekend. I did! I started having contractions within 24 hours of discontinuing the terbulatine and Katherine Elsie was born on 4 August, Sunday, weighing a healthy 6lb, 15½oz by C-section. I was able to hold her within a couple of hours after she was born. I unwrapped her, counted her toes and fingers and held her 'kangaroo care' style for hours as I slept.

She has been perfectly healthy—I was able to actually enjoy her first year. However, Katherine is a real free spirit. The tantrums that child threw! WOW! Kaia tried to imitate her sister when she was about 3 years old. She lay down on the floor, spread her arms wide and said "Mum, I'm angry!" I just smiled down at her and said "You forgot to scream." She got up, dusted off her trousers and smiled at me. She never tried it again. I found out later that year that Kaia was short for Katherine in Norwegian. As they get older, I have noticed how ironic this is. They are as close as identical twins, but as different as night and day. Just like their names!

The doctor who delivered Katherine suggested, after she was born, that I shouldn't have any more children. I was heartbroken AND relieved. My husband always wanted eight! The doctor said that I hadn't healed well from my first C-section and delivering Katherine had been very difficult with all of the scar tissue. It would be nearly impossible for him to deliver another baby safely. I was also told that I would never be able to deliver vaginally because I have a heart-shaped uterus (called a bicornuate uterus), which allows the baby only half the space to grow and no space in which to turn near the end of the pregnancy. (This had no affect on Kaia being born prematurely, incidentally.)

Today, both of my children are healthy and happy. They are the lights of my life. I know I wouldn't be the person I am today without the experiences of having them and bringing them up. They have taught me so much and made me stronger. I am forever grateful. Thank you, baby girls! I love you!

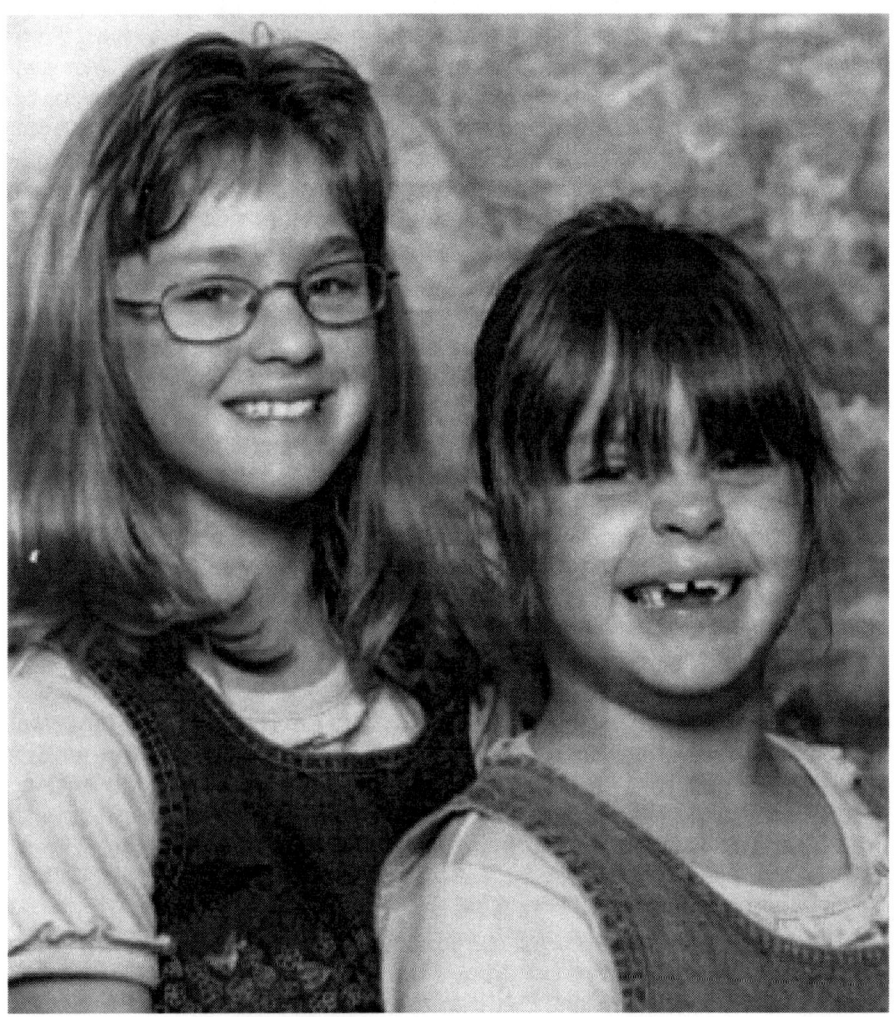

Kaia, aged 8, with her sister Katherine, aged 7

Overcoming bad first experiences...

I must admit, the reason I started writing about birth and collecting birth stories was because of all the bad experiences I'd heard about. Again and again, I met women whose births had 'gone wrong' for some reason or another. My conclusion—after much reflection and many interrogations of women I met at baby groups, playgroups, in the street, *anywhere*—was that they'd had bad experiences basically because of a lack of preparation of one kind or another. (The book *Preparing for a Healthy Birth* goes into this in detail.) On the plus side, though, I did meet many women who learnt from a bad first experience and then went on to have very successful second and subsequent births, often with the help and support of excellent midwives...

Better luck next time...

Pauline Farrance and Michael White

The mother's account:

I sat down to write about the wonder of Rosie's birth at home, but felt it all started over two years ago with Sean's birth in hospital, which affected both myself and my family so much that we were determined our next baby's introduction to our world would be a happier and easier event. So, firstly, I am writing about the birth of Sean Henry, our first child.

I attended excellent NCT antenatal classes, which helped me to look forward with excitement to my baby's arrival, instead of with the fear of childbirth which I'd always held. I had hoped for a natural and gentle birth but due to slightly raised blood pressure following a family crisis, at 36 weeks I found myself on the local hospital baby extraction line. Although I instinctively and intellectually felt that all the intervention was unnecessary and indeed dangerous, and that the baby was the best judge of when he would be 'better out than in' (the antenatal ward catchphrase), I did not have the confidence to totally resist the daily pressure from the doctors during my two weeks on the ward. Being told I was killing my baby did not help the situation—or my blood pressure!—although some of the midwives were very kind and supportive and were obviously concerned at the number of inductions being performed. However, I did have the knowledge and courage to decline their frequent offers to break my waters (at 1cm dilation) and 'pop' me down to the theatre for a nice, convenient, planned caesarean.

Unfortunately, due to the constant harassment and worry, my blood pressure rose even higher and I finally agreed to prostaglandin pessaries and had seven inserted over seven days. Sean still showed no sign of budging, which simply meant that he was not ready for the outside world. (All my other tests on urine and placenta, etc were perfectly normal.) I was then a Failed Induction and subjected to the full panoply of modern obstetrics: waters broken, numerous drips (including syntocinon), gas and air, and meptid. I didn't really know what was going on during 15 hours of labour, except that everything stopped at one point—not surprising with that cocktail of drugs, which made me quite unable to stray from the bed.

The resultant birth was a 'normal delivery' with a bullying, insensitive midwife who took Sean away immediately (despite my written and oral requests to the contrary) and returned him to me clean and swaddled, so that I couldn't even get to see or touch his fingers. I didn't have a chance to put him to the breast for four hours, despite frequent requests for help, and Sean and I had great difficulty with feeding for ages afterwards. He was sleepy for a few days due to the drugs he received through me and I was in such a state trying to fend off the bottles from the night staff, it is amazing we ever got the hang of breastfeeding! Needless to say, it took me nearly a year to get over the trauma of those three weeks, so when Mike and I found we were expecting another baby, we realised that we could not risk the same things happening again, especially as I would have to be on top form to cope with a baby and our extremely boisterous 2-year-old.

The reactions of the medical profession to my request for a home birth could take me through several paragraphs. Suffice to say, it made everyone very twitchy. Tactics used to dissuade me ranged from coercion to disbelief ("There is no such thing as a home birth in this country") and from the usual threats ("What if something should go wrong?") to the sudden discovery of a problem with my antibodies which meant the baby should be checked by a paediatrician at birth!... none of which, of course, were valid.

I pursued every avenue imaginable and pestered all sorts of people in my determination to ensure that this time my baby and I would not start off our relationship emotionally battered. Time was running out when I read an article in the newspaper about Michel Odent. It appeared that he had attended some home births, so I attempted to contact him via his publisher. A few days later I answered the phone to a gentle French accent—I couldn't believe my luck. Much to our amazement, Michel was willing to attend our baby's birth if possible (he refused to use the word 'deliver'). From then on we just hoped the baby would have the good sense to be born out of rush hour times as we knew that, with Michel, we would be able to truly get to know our new baby during that very sensitive period immediately after the birth and she would be treated with gentleness and respect.

The big event: I wake up on 9 October feeling that this would be a good day to have a baby—the sun is shining and I feel well and reasonably energetic for a change. Baby due today, though, so I'm sure nothing will happen. Cathy and daughter Emily (aged 2) are coming to have lunch and spend the afternoon with us.

Around mid morning I feel very mild period-type pains but I had them Friday night so I take no notice. About 1.30pm I have to stop for a moment through the quickening—I couldn't really describe it as a pain—but manage to prepare a simple lunch quite easily. We sit down to lunch about 2.00pm and I finally tell Cathy that I am having 'pains' but think it is probably a false alarm. About an hour later Mike comes in from painting the gates outside to have lunch and I tell him about the 'pains'. He says he'll finish the gates but I tell him I'd rather he didn't risk welcoming our baby into the world covered in black gloss. It then registers that something might really be happening so he looks a bit panicky and rushes about in confusion.

4.00pm: I still can't be convinced I'm definitely in labour as I'm not really in pain and I don't want to call Michel unless I'm sure, so we start writing down times. Contractions seem to be about three minutes apart. Mike gets electric fires and polythene sheets (the only special equipment needed) and looks agitated. I keep laughing because I can't believe this is the real thing. Everything is so normal and Sean is rushing about terrorising Emily, as usual.

4.40pm: Mike decides it's time to call Michel—he's getting worried about being 'in charge', I think. Luck is with us and he is at home and says he will be right over. Cathy sits reading a book with Sean and Emily and I join in, but have to stop suddenly to lean on the back of the chair. Emily asks, "What's Auntie Pauline doing?" "Having a baby, darling". We both can't stop laughing, which is a bit tricky during a contraction. My own sensitive little angel hasn't noticed a thing!

5.30pm: Cathy prepares food for the children as Mike is not capable in present state of agitation. I go upstairs to change but keep getting delayed by a contraction. It's cool and peaceful upstairs and contractions seem stronger.

5.40pm: Mike is looking out of the window and announces Michel's arrival with great relief. I greet him with a smile then wish I hadn't as he tells me I don't look like a woman in labour. We show him our list of times of contractions but he isn't interested. (Michel told us that he can tell if labour is normal and how it is progressing simply by listening to the noises an uninhibited woman makes and I remember clearly how I could not stop myself from making different noises as labour got stronger.)

5.50pm: I go upstairs with Michel and he checks baby's heart and my blood pressure as I tell him it has been raised... in fact to the same level as when I was admitted with Sean. It's now the lowest it's been for two weeks.

6.00pm: Children having tea with Cathy. Michel joins them to chat to Cathy and asks about their bedtime. (He had previously told us that it is best not to have anyone else around for the birth as the number of people present is directly proportional to the length of labour, and the longer the labour the more likely complications occur.) Mike orders pizzas for himself and Michel due to vivid recollection of no food or drink for 12 hours before Sean's birth and we feel it will be a long night.

6.45pm: Cathy and Emily leave. Mike takes Sean up to bed—skips the bath today! Pizzas arrive.

7.00pm: Sean asleep in record time. Contractions getting stronger now. I try out the newly acquired bean bag but it radiates heat back at me so I kneel in front of the sofa with my head on my arms, leaning on the seat, swaying my hips through contractions. I had intended to wear my 'Singapore happy coat' for the birth but don't feel like moving now! It is incredible how the contractions have taken off now it is quiet and there are no distractions. Mike has organised our birthing music—Irish harp and music from a band called 'Clannad', which is very soothing.

7.15pm: Contractions stronger so I start moaning through them. Mike and Michel chomping away on pizzas at the other end of the room. Mike comes over to see how I am and reminds me to 'breathe', which I had forgotten! He gets me a pillow to lean on which is lovely and cool. I ask him to hurry and finish his pizza as I'm in pain!

7.25pm: Making a lot of noise now as contractions really hurt and I'm worried about coping for hours like this. I hear Mike make a move to get up but Michel whispers that I am best left 'in my own world'. Any outside interference will delay things.

7.30pm: Mike now joins me. He is very calm and reassuring and I hold him through contractions.

7.45pm: I feel I want to go to the toilet. I remember this feeling before Sean was born but don't allow myself to possibly imagine baby is coming as I couldn't bear the disappointment if it's a false alarm. Mike helps me upstairs between contractions. I sit on the toilet and feel very constipated and confused. Waters break. Maybe baby is coming... I put my hand down thinking I might feel the head and find blood on my hand. Michel comes upstairs and tells Mike to get the electric fires on at the bathroom door—we have a very small bathroom!—so we know this must be IT. Mike helps me off the toilet and they pull my clothes off and Michel tells him to hold me from behind in the supported squat. I feel my uterus push and a burning sensation and give a little cry as (at 7.55pm) baby's head is born. Then my uterus pushes again. Mike and I are still standing in suspended animation as Michel tells us to look down at our baby daughter lying in his hands! We can't believe she has arrived so quickly and easily. Michel hands her to me and I cradle our beautiful daughter in my arms, her lovely virgin skin touching mine. The wonder and joy of that moment, to be holding my newborn babe so close and feeling her perfect little body next to mine, I can never describe. I kept saying to Mike "We have a little girl!" and his face was alight with happiness.

I sat in the bathroom amidst the goo and mess for about 30 minutes while Michel and Mike sorted things out. I was blissfully unaware of what was going on, having eyes only for my baby. I remember Michel tying the cord after about 10 minutes and Mike cut it and found it quite tough! Then Mike took Rose Eleanor while I went to lie on the bed.

About 9.00pm Michel felt my stomach and said the placenta had separated. He massaged my stomach and the placenta came away with a contraction. Mike was trying to clear up the bathroom and was pleased the birth hadn't been on a carpet! Michel left about 10.00pm and we sat in bed marvelling at our new baby daughter. She was very alert and never cried, although she gave the occasional whimper. We had the lights very low for her all the time. She didn't want to suck immediately after the birth but kept nuzzling my breast and looking around. Mike opened a bottle of champagne but I didn't like to drink more than a glass so I contented myself with two packets of Mintolas! We sat and caressed our little miracle and talked over and over about her birth, we were both so excited. About 2.00am I thought we should get some sleep and maybe Rose Eleanor was tired, so we all snuggled up in our bed. It was incredible that Sean had slept through all this but at 5.00am he woke and came into our bed. His little face was a picture when he heard Rosie stirring and he laughed and said "Baby sister!"—he was so happy to see her.

The father's tale:

Whenever there was a choice I have always opted for nature's way in areas such as food, environment and general health. However, this had never extended to having a baby and I preferred to abdicate the responsibility to the medical profession, who appeared more than willing to take over.

I attended the NCT classes and that's when doubts began to creep in, especially as I learnt of all the medical hardware, paraphernalia and drugs that were deemed essential nowadays for giving birth. I began to realise that the medical profession was perhaps, after all, just as horrified as I at having the responsibility for the birth.

However, we went ahead with the hospital birth of our firstborn as it was decided by a hospital screening process that Pauline's blood pressure was outside the norm, for which she was immediately admitted. Sean was eventually extracted in a very workmanlike manner, some two and a half weeks of protestations, seven pessaries, two gas tanks, two doses of chemicals, 10 yards of graph paper, one cup of tea and 15 hours of narcotic trance later. It would be an understatement to say it was a very traumatic time for all of us and I was disappointed at not experiencing the joy one has heard about as the father in attendance at the birth of his first child. It was more a sense of overwhelming relief that the whole episode was over with and all three parties (physically) healthy and alive.

This time we were determined from the outset that this baby would be born at home so we could have more control and responsibility

16 months later we found we were expecting our second baby and this time we were determined from the outset that this baby would be born at home so that we could have more control and responsibility. Our GP reluctantly agreed to cover the birth but opposition grew from all quarters of the medical profession and eventually no doctor would agree to cover the birth at home. This again I would attribute to their horror at having the responsibility for the birth. However, in desperation and clutching at any possible straw, Pauline managed to meet Michel Odent, who agreed to be present at the birth, if he was available.

The day of the birth thankfully arrived on a Sunday. Although we had read every possible piece of literature on the subject, I was filled with dread and my heart began to palpitate. I thought I might possibly have to deliver the baby myself if Michel was held up in the traffic... I began to race around looking for textbooks, plastic sheets and the bucket. (The requirement for the bucket had somehow lodged in my mind from the NCT course.)

I began to race around looking for textbooks, plastic sheets and the bucket

I was greatly relieved when a French-registered Renault pulled up outside and the calming presence of Michel entered the house. I had by this time got my act together and put on some soothing music. Later, we turned the lights down very low and Michel told me to let Pauline get into her own world. We chatted casually as we ate the enormous home delivery pizzas while Pauline got on with the business of having a baby, leaning on the sofa with her head in a pillow. For some reason I was convinced it would be a long night and I was building up my reserves of energy in anticipation! Minutes after finishing the pizzas we were all in our tiny bathroom with me holding Pauline in the supported squat and Michel holding a beautiful baby girl in his hands. She gave what seemed to be an obligatory whimper to let us know she was OK and settled blissfully into her mother's arms and there they stayed for about half an hour. I was totally dumbstruck by the ease and beauty of the birth and just gazed in disbelief. After coming back down to Earth, I began clearing up operations and gave thanks for lino tiles instead of carpet in the bathroom, but wished I hadn't eaten the pizza! Michel's presence was quite unobtrusive throughout his visit, but it was his confidence and experience in allowing nature to take its course without any unnecessary interference which made the birth such a trouble-free and memorable event, and gave us so much joy and confidence during the weeks that followed.

We have talked endlessly about the birth and were so happy and grateful that everything had gone so well, but we felt so sad for the vast majority of mothers (and fathers) who are denied the joy of such a precious and unique experience in our so-called civilised society today. It is widely accepted that about 90% of women are able to give birth normally, without complications, so why don't we keep the costly expertise and machinery for those who really need it? Of course, many men and women are happier in the hospital environment and we would never try and dissuade them from this as the labour will always be prolonged by fear and anxiety. But the present day fear of complications during childbirth is largely unfounded and we should look at the event in perspective as a part of family life.

We were so excited by Rosie's birth that we were on a high for at least a week and had loads of energy to carry us through the sleepless nights, etc. Added benefits of the birth at home include much less disruption and confusion for older brothers and sisters and it meant so much to my parents to be able to hold their second grandchild so soon after she was born—a privilege not allowed after Sean's birth. In addition, the baby will not succumb to any of the infections which abound in hospital.

To put it all in a nutshell, three days after Rosie's birth we were feeling a little down because we had enjoyed the birth so much. We wanted the clock to turn back to Sunday so that we could do it all again!

Rushing home from hospital

Jennifer Jacoby

The birth of my first child felt very institutionalised and governed by hospital policy. The midwife was definitely in control of the entire situation with me as her charge. My second birth was a truly wonderful experience that was influenced by an extremely intuitive midwife who encouraged me to do what I felt to be right for me. These experiences have made me highly aware of the dynamics between the birthing mother and the midwife whose main purpose is to provide support for the mother and her partner in labour and who needs to understand both the physical processes and the emotional needs of the mother. I feel that this relationship is one of the most important factors during labour and birth.

In my second pregnancy, when I was fairly overdue, I decided to try acupuncture on Wednesday evening to get my labour started. That night I was woken at about 2.00am with fairly mild contractions but they had completely fizzled out by 6.00am. My husband took Thursday off work as we were hoping that something might happen. I had woken him up at 4.00am to put the TENS machine on me, which I found to be more annoying than helpful.

I found the TENS machine more annoying than helpful

I had been convinced throughout my pregnancy that my labour would be very short and worried that my husband wouldn't make it home in time for the birth as we live in North Finchley and he works at Bart's hospital in Smithfield. Of course nothing happened that day and we went to bed on Thursday evening thoroughly disappointed.

I had had irate hospital staff phoning me all week and harassing me because I was refusing to go and see a consultant to talk about induction. We had planned a home birth and had hired a birthing pool and I was really looking forward to it. I had started to feel somewhat despondent and felt that my whole labour and birthing experience was about to be taken over by hospital staff. I reluctantly agreed to go to the Barnet General on Friday morning to be monitored and see a consultant, as I didn't think anyone would try and induce me then and there and wouldn't be rushed into any decisions as I would have the weekend to think any choices over.

I was woken up at 2.00am on Friday morning with mild contractions and slept in between them until 4.00am when I felt I had to get up and move around. I spent the early hours of the morning walking around the garden and tidying bits and pieces in the house. I woke my husband at 6.00am and we played Scrabble for an hour and then phoned the midwife at 7.00am to say we wouldn't be going to the hospital that morning as my contractions had started up again. She phoned back half an hour later to say she would come and visit us on her way into work.

By the time the midwife arrived (at 9.30am) my contractions had stopped. She stayed with us for about 40 minutes and just before she left I had a fairly mild contraction. She asked me to go to the hospital to be monitored and we agreed and set off at about 10.30 with my first daughter, Milly (aged 2).

We arrived at Barnet General Hospital and I was monitored in the Day Unit. Although my contractions had started up again (at seven-minute intervals) they were relatively mild and not getting closer together. I thought they were probably Braxton Hicks contractions as I was beginning to think this baby was never going to be born.

The consultant came to see me at 1.00pm and booked me in for an induction the following Friday because he only does inductions on a Friday. As he was talking he looked at me and asked if I was OK. I replied that I was fine, just having a contraction. He wanted to know why no one had told him I was in labour and I told him I wasn't but I was just having very mild contractions. He wanted to examine me, which he did. I knew something was up by the look on his face and then he said "If you want a home birth you had better get in the car and hurry because you are 5cm dilated and your waters are bulging." It seemed as though a cheer went up with all the midwives in the Day Unit and everyone, including us, was excited, not to mention surprised. One of the midwives phoned my midwife to get her to meet us at home and I dressed, got our things together and hurried back to the car.

Before you start to think that I have an incredible pain threshold you should be aware that the contractions I had with the birth of my first daughter were started artificially with syntocinon and were so incredibly painful (as any unlucky person who has had it can tell you). These were the only comparison of contractions I had.

We got home at 1.30pm and my husband put Milly to bed (very quickly) and then set about filling the birthing pool we had hired. I got the baby's clothes, etc ready, phoned my mother-in-law to come round and look after Milly and then phoned my mum in Australia and a couple of friends to let them know my pregnancy was finally coming to an end. My midwife arrived at 2.15pm and just after that my contractions got serious. The pool was ready at 3.00pm and I got into it. Throughout the whole experience I was amazed with the role the midwife took, as it was so different to my last birthing experience in hospital. She didn't examine me internally and only monitored the baby about three or four times. I kept asking what I should be doing and every time she replied "What do you feel like doing?"

Rosa was born under the water at 4.11pm weighing in at 9lb 4oz (4.2 kg). I had a small tear along my episiotomy scar that didn't require stitches. By 6.00pm all the family had arrived (truck loads of them) and we were all downstairs singing 'Happy Birthday' to Rosa and eating birthday cake. Rosa is now 11 weeks old and is the most peaceful, relaxed baby I have ever known. She has always slept well (probably due to her incredible size) but now a bad night's sleep for Rosa is sleeping from 9.00pm to 6.30am. The midwife who delivered Rosa works out of Barnet General Hospital and is proof that a terrific midwife makes all the difference. I can't even begin to describe how fantastic she was! We owe our perfect birth experience to her expertise.

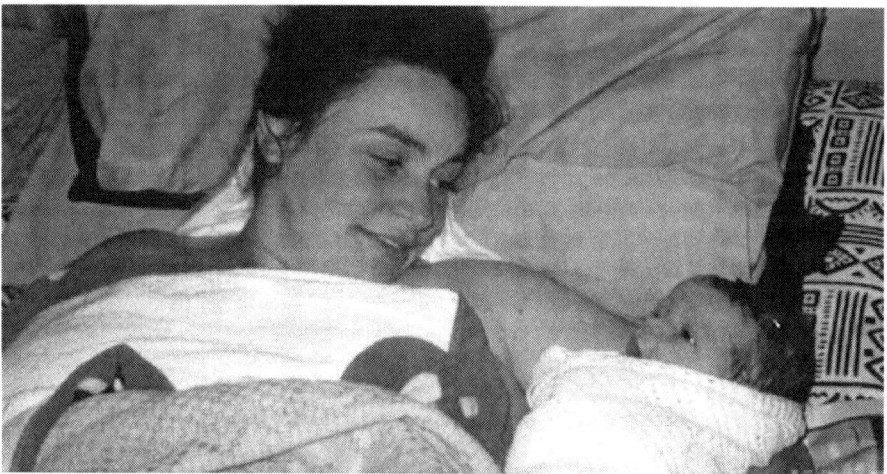

Jennifer with baby Rosa, just after the birth

A more relaxed second and third time

Christina Mansi

I had my first child, Samantha, in January 1985 but what influenced my expectations and hopes was a TV programme I'd watched about four years before. The programme had Miriam Stoppard as its hostess and the subject was Michel Odent and his work in Pithiviers, France as a natural childbirth pioneer. It inspired me to read books about the subject (home births, natural birth—by Sheila Kitzinger and Michel Odent) and my enthusiasm grew. When I first became pregnant I sought out a doctor who was sympathetic and experienced, who would attend me at home.

I sought out a doctor who was sympathetic

The labour started on Saturday morning. The first sign was a little gush of amniotic fluid—but no pain. The doctor examined me, and assessed that I was not dilated at all. He seemed a bit put out that this was happening on a Saturday—he had to visit his sick wife in hospital. I tried the usual tricks to bring the labour on—taking castor oil and scrubbing floors.

The doctor said at 3.30pm that we had better go to hospital as some hours had elapsed since the waters had leaked; he said that there was a risk of infection and that the baby could become blind if that happened. We went to the hospital very disappointed and frightened. The house doctor at the hospital read the letter of introduction from my 'home birth doctor' (who had to go to visit his wife). He looked and acted very disdainfully towards me—that I'd hoped for a home birth and now here I was needing professional help after all. I was wired up to a machine to measure contractions... there were none. I'd heard about the method called sweeping the cervix whereby the doctor uses his fingers to manipulate the cervix into loosening, and maybe rupturing the membranes. I wanted to try this first before resorting to drugs. It was done very painfully and some contractions started.

Over the hours, I was put on a syntocinon drip—the contractions were not strong enough and the baby had to be delivered within 12 hours, according to the hospital's rule, because of the risk of infection. I had the water sac broken so that a monitor could be attached to the baby's head. This was very upsetting and painful. I felt raped. So much water came out—I realised that before it was only a leak and was not as dangerous for infection as the full water emptying. Then I was persuaded to have an epidural because they wanted to increase the syntocinon to speed things up. The baby's pulse was now dropping so low they were worried, so they phoned their top doctor who advised a caesarean. The epidural was wearing off now and I could feel the baby low down in the canal, almost ready to come out. They still went ahead with a general anaesthetic and I woke up to see my husband showing my lovely baby wrapped up tight in a shawl. She was born at 12.30am, nine hours after I went to the hospital.

I was so happy to have a lovely baby that I soon forgot about my ordeal. On Samantha's first birthday I relived the humiliating, disappointing and painful time of her birth. I duly wrote a letter to the hospital. I complained about my treatment. I did receive a reply and I was invited to meet the doctors at the hospital for a talk/discussion. I did not go in the end as I felt that I would be out of my depth at the meeting—and it would be me against them. I had already been through a lot of grief with Samantha's health since she was 8 months old. A doctor at the hospital had told me she had a heart murmur. She was also taking a paediatric steroid in tablet form to try to combat the low blood count they had discovered she had because of a rare blood disease called Diamond Blackfan anaemia. I had enough battles to win ahead of me. I discovered that a suggested allergy to wheat could be her problem. We discovered that in fact her blood count went up when she didn't eat wheat or other wheat gluten products. It took me three years to finally wean her off steroids. She's now a healthy young lady, though.

My second labour started in the same way...

My second daughter, Kathryn, was born in February 1988. I made contact with Michel Odent, who was living in London then. I wanted to try again for a home birth and he agreed to help and support me.

The first sign of labour was a gush of amniotic fluid, as before. This was at 8.30pm. The real labour pains came at 10.30pm. Kathryn was born on my bed at 2.30am after four hours of labour. It was painful and I was glad to be on my own in the dark of my bedroom. My husband and Michel Odent were there but kept out of the way and didn't interfere.

At the last moment Michel Odent came over and helped, while my husband supported me under the arms as I gave birth in a supported squat position. She weighed 7lb 2oz. I held Kathryn immediately and put her to my breast. About half an hour later the afterbirth was expelled naturally.

I was in shock for the first half hour after Kathryn's birth and was shivering—but that is apparently normal—so we turned on the electric fan heater. Kathryn did not cry when she was born. She lay on my thighs—skin-to-skin—for a long time, contentedly looking around in the half light. I breastfed Kathryn exclusively (no solids) until she was 6-8 months old. I didn't have my first period until she was 18 months old and carried on feeding her until two months before my third child was born, when she was 2 years 4 months.

My son Anthony was born in August 1990. I had put on more weight with this pregnancy than before. He was overdue by a week or so. We had visitors—relatives—staying in our home at the time. The night that the guests went to spend one night away my labour started at 10.30pm. It was a long and hard labour—six hours. The second stage only really started when I forced myself to get up into a squatting position.

Michel Odent, who had been outside the room listening to the progress of my labour, came in as I was starting to push. He helped to deliver Anthony's shoulders. He later said that his shoulders were broad—he was a bigger baby than the others: 8lb 4oz. I recovered quickly again and breastfed him until my second son (my fourth child) Jonathan was born in October '92.

Jonathan was four weeks' overdue. My labour started at 8.30pm and he was born at 10.30pm. I wanted to try a water birth so I was in my extra large bath with lots of lavender oil when the midwife arrived at 9.30pm. (Michel Odent was not in the country at the time.) She didn't think that I was in real labour as I seemed so calm in the water. When I got out of the bath to call her from my bedroom she was surprised. Jonathan was born on the floor of the bathroom, my husband again helping to support me in a squat position. I had no tears, he didn't look overdue and weighed 7lb 14oz. I breastfed him till he was over 3. I felt very emotional when I tried to stop. He was my last baby. He's now 9 years old!

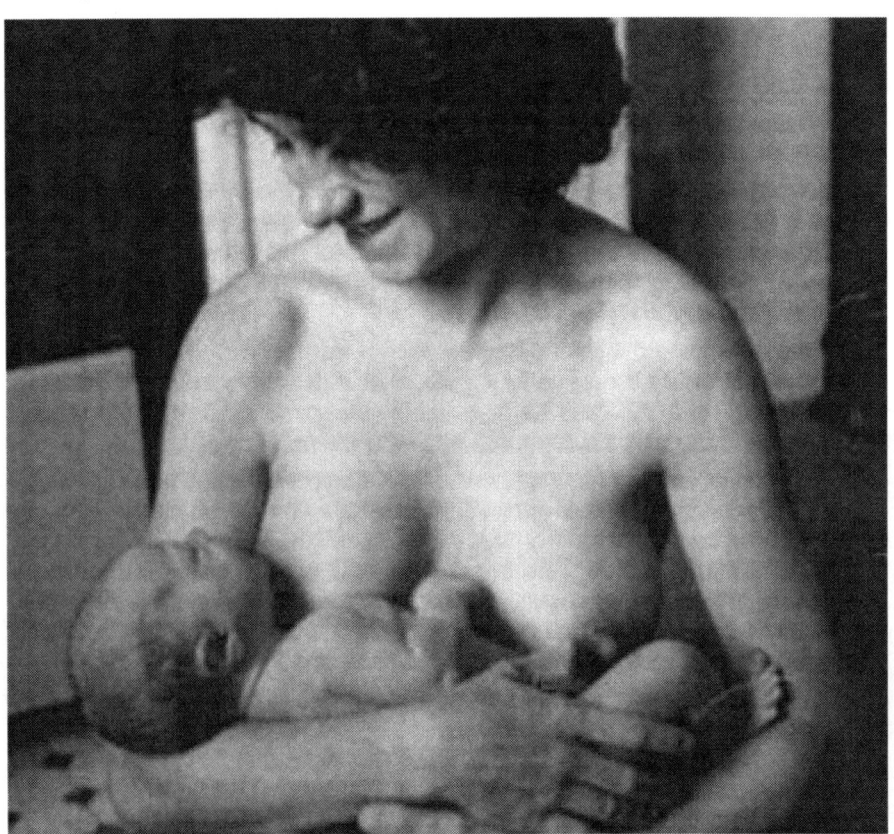

Liliana (see right) cradling one of her newborn babies
Photo © Jill Furmanovsky

You're being watched!

Liliana Lammers

When expecting my first child, I registered at a London hospital, as the most natural thing to do... I was born in hospital... and my mother too! It was 1983, I arrived smiling and I was told, after an internal, that I was 8cm. One hour later I found myself in a labour ward, surrounded by 10 students, a male doctor and a midwife, and a monstrous fetal monitoring machine was attached to me and sounding very loud. Bright lights, voices everywhere, people coming in and out, my partner at my right... I was soon in a state of shock. Labour almost came to an end. Epidural, episiotomy and a very light and unnecessary forceps followed. "Never again. Never again", I kept repeating to myself, while holding my baby daughter.

> "Never again. Never again," I kept repeating to myself, while holding my baby daughter

In 1987 I was expecting for the second time. I kept well away from doctors, hospitals and all their machinery. I was feeling wonderful—I knew my baby was well. I wanted to stay at home this time. A friend of mine mentioned Michel Odent... I read a bit about him... "Yes, he will understand me." He did. I had the most beautiful, undisturbed birth one can possibly imagine. Another daughter.

And two years later my son was born. Big boy, 9lb 8oz. Born between lunch and pudding! Literally. I was so lucky to be assisted by Michel Odent again.

> Big boy... born between lunch and pudding!

I was in labour but very hungry, to everyone's surprise. I had a big lunch and then, when the cake I had baked that morning was approaching the kitchen table, I stood up suddenly and with an unusually loud voice said "No pudding. The baby's coming!"—and, turning to my partner: "Do the washing up." After this, I rushed into a dark room I had prepared, went on my knees, on the floor, burying my head in pillows.

One and a half hours later I was lying down on the floor, my baby on my chest, both warmly wrapped, the cord not yet cut... and eating the cake! (This child is now 17 and has always had an incredible appetite.)

My fourth child was born at dawn, in a friend's sitting room, at a time when I could only hear the birds singing... and Michel Odent gently sleeping at the other end of the room. It was so magical, sweet, beautiful. My baby girl found the breast in minutes!

> My fourth child was born at dawn in a friend's sitting room when I could only hear the birds singing

Getting the right support

Liz Woolley

I have had two breech babies. The first, a boy, was born in 1999 by caesarean, the second, a girl, was born naturally in 2001.

I was a breech baby and so was my brother, so it shouldn't have been a surprise when it became clear that my second child had no intention of turning round, but I kept thinking she would. I tried external cephalic version (ECV) and moxabustion, as well as lots of undignified bum-in-the-air positions. But as nothing was working, my midwife and I began to plan for a breech birth.

My midwife and I began to prepare for a breech birth...

With my first baby, I had encountered a lot of opposition to having my son vaginally at the hospital where I was registered. As he only turned breech a few days before my due date, I had little opportunity to find any alternatives, let alone research whether what I was being told about risks was accurate. After he was born by caesarean I felt very upset emotionally, as well as physically. Obviously, I was happy to have him, but I felt 'all wrong'. I had gone into labour and then had an emergency section and my body felt strange, literally as though it was still pent up, still had something left to do. I can't explain it in words. I felt like I had let my body down and let my baby down.

Second time around I had an independent midwife, Judith, with lots of experience of breech birth and had also switched hospitals and booked with a consultant who was prepared to support my efforts for a vaginal birth. Both Judith and the consultant felt that the studies on breech birth had not given enough weight to the impact different skills and experience of midwives/ doctors had in determining outcomes. However, we were all clear that whilst we were trying for a breech birth, at any sign of problems we would go straight for a caesarean. Given this and the small risk of a problem with my previous section, we felt we had to opt for a hospital birth.

A couple of days before my due date, my waters broke as I was cooking the evening meal. There were no contractions so we went ahead with our dinner with my partner's brother, who then took our son to his grandparents. I phoned Judith, who called round to test if it was definitely amniotic fluid. I was happy for her to leave while we awaited developments. At about 10.00pm I started having contractions. They were anything from 10 to two minutes apart and quite strong. In between, I tried to read to keep calm. We wrote down times. Past midnight I was sick a few times and my partner managed to doze off for a bit. As it approached 6.00am I decided I wanted to leave for the hospital. Although it's only about 12 miles away, I wanted to beat the terrible rush-hour traffic jams.

Judith met us at the door of the hospital. Walking brought contractions thick and fast; I had one in the three yards between car and door, one in the elevator and a couple in the corridor. We went into a large room with a long row of windows, giving a good view over the city—we were four floors up. I said to Judith that after a whole night of contractions the last thing I needed was to be told I was only 2cm dilated. She said, "Shall we not look then?" So we didn't.

For a long time, I crouched on the floor and held on to a metal chair leg with each contraction, staring intently at the pattern on the hard tiles. After a while, Judith said she wanted me to get things moving by walking about more. With her on one side and my partner on the other we processed up and down the long room, lifting our feet up as high as we could. As before, walking brought a rush of strong contractions.

At around midday Judith examined me and pronounced me 6-7cm dilated— good job she hadn't checked earlier. We kept walking but I refused to leave the room to take to the corridors. We had been left completely alone by the hospital staff and I couldn't bear the idea of seeing anyone else. Every now and then I was sick. As the afternoon wore on, Judith started getting me holding the end of the bed, squatting and imagining the baby moving down. At this stage, I don't think I actually believed that this baby would really be born and be born through my efforts.

Another examination showed that I was almost fully dilated. Judith quietly told me that the next part would be very hard work, but that if I wanted an epidural I could still do that. Having done so much already, I felt determined not to do this and risk the interventions that could follow. I told her I was scared of what was to come. She said being scared would make it harder, so I decided not to be. It seems incredible that you can decide not to be scared, but that is what I seemed to do.

I was very hot and sweaty and Judith suggested changing clothes. Once I got my big T-shirt off, I refused to put another one on. It felt like it would be a distraction. Judith told me to start pushing with contractions. I couldn't get the hang of it at all. I felt no urge to push, I felt like I was pretending. I tried to think about a beautiful baby coming down. After a while I started to understand that I needed to push really hard and for a long time each time. I think the penny finally dropped that it was really up to me to do this and that I would have to work harder than I believed possible.

Judith said she could tell what sex the baby was (a quirk of having a breech). Then, after a big push, I finally felt the baby moving through me. I was leaning over the back of the chair when another push brought the baby's bottom out. I shouted to Judith as I was scared the baby would drop out onto the floor. The consultant was now in the room. She, my midwife and partner all lifted me onto the bed. This felt awful as it felt like the baby was being pushed back inside. Judith said to me: "The more of this you can do yourself the better."

The next contraction I gave a big push and the legs came out; the next brought the arms and shoulders spinning out.

Then there was what felt like a very long silent moment. I could see the sunset through the big windows. I could see the midwife and consultant looking at me. I wondered if they were worried, if there was a time limit on this bit. I didn't wait for a contraction but decided to push with all my might, to get the baby's head out as quickly as I could. Then she was in my arms. A bit blue but soon pink, not crying, very calm, big eyes open in the dimly lit room as night began to fall.

I felt a bit sore for about half an hour and then felt fine. Physically and emotionally I felt great then and for about three days afterwards. Really great, super-happy, full of energy. I awoke each morning with what felt like a hangover. Judith said it was coming down from the endorphins. Partly, I felt great too because I was amazingly proud of myself. I had no pain relief, no interventions and no stitches and a breech baby! Particularly after having a section for breech position the first time around, it seemed almost incredible.

The experience of a vaginal birth

Nina Klose

My mother says that newborns look like little angels that haven't fully descended to Earth yet. Newborns do have a faraway look in their eyes. But if you've given birth, you'd hardly say they come from the sky. There is nothing ethereal about pushing a baby into the world. It is just the opposite, a wholly carnal and earthy experience. Pushing out my daughter felt like doing a very large and difficult poo out my vagina.

People keep telling me I had an easy labour. I'm sure it was, relatively speaking. Now that it's over, I'd be ready to do it again next week. But it didn't feel easy. It hurt like anything. The thing is, I was so thrilled that my body was doing what it needed to do, that I hardly minded the pain. With our first child I never went into established labour. During his birth, I had had fairly regular, painful contractions from early in the morning, but labour never became 'well established', according to the midwives who examined me.

It's hard to pinpoint exactly what went wrong. Was it because I hadn't fully visualised what it meant for the fetus to descend through my pelvis and out into the world? That I couldn't see myself becoming a mother? Was it because I allowed the doctors to 're-date' my pregnancy based on the 12-week scan, even though I *knew* when I had conceived? They pushed the official due date two weeks earlier. This made me more anxious about being induced, so I tried to initiate the labour with nipple stimulation early in the morning of the day my labour started. Maybe trying to induce was the starting point of the problems. Maybe he hadn't got into the right position and wasn't quite ready to be born yet. My waters broke at 6.00am. I phoned the birth centre, but since nobody asked me, I never mentioned to the midwife that my waters had broken. I figured, since they didn't ask, it couldn't be important. I was in what I thought was labour all day long but we only went to the birth centre in the evening. I discovered a light green blush of fresh meconium on my sanitary towel. But I had just changed the pad so when I got there—a long drive all the way across town—the midwives didn't believe me and sent me home. I phoned again when we got back—I was sure it was meconium. We drove back, this time in the small hours. The birth centre confirmed that it was meconium and sent me straight back across town again to the hospital. Hospital staff were unsympathetic to my desire for a normal, unmedicated birth.

I will never forget the calm before the storm, the two hours' respite they agreed to give us before starting an induction. My contractions had ceased entirely. I stood at the window of the hospital praying for the labour to resume. My womb was still resting as the sun rose. I realised I would soon be forced to acquiesce to the hospital's interventions. I requested an epidural before the induction... but no one told me that the chances of a C-section are over five times higher with an epidural! (Isn't there a legal requirement to inform patients about the risks they face??) The baby couldn't tolerate the heavy spasms of induced contractions. His heart-rate plummeted. They turned off the drip. His heart rate settled. But there were still no effective contractions, the waters had been broken for over 24 hours and I had not dilated past a few centimetres. If I had been at home, I probably would have gone calmly to sleep, rested up and then given birth. Or perhaps he was in a funny position. Who knows? The doctor who delivered him couldn't find any clear explanation for the meconium or why he hadn't descended.

For me, agreeing to the caesarean felt like a death sentence. I had so longed to give my son a good birth and to experience that life-changing moment of pushing him into the world. Why did the caesarean have to happen? I still ask myself. If I had it to do over again, I believe the most important problem was no continuity of care. If I'd been attended by one midwife throughout the pregnancy and birth, I'm sure I wouldn't have felt pressured into trying to induce the birth. And everything might have been different.

Technically, my second labour took only five hours early Thursday morning, from when the first strong contractions began after midnight, until the placenta was born around 5.00am. But I'd call it a 10-hour labour with a day's break in the middle. I was awake most of Tuesday night with contractions every 10 minutes that were strong enough to get me out of bed but not strong enough to have to shout and holler. I sat up on the sofa and breathed hard until about 6.00am when they started to ease off.

"I'm in labour!" I announced proudly to my midwife on Wednesday morning. "I told my husband he could stay home from work. Was that the right thing to do?" "You're not in labour and he has to go to work," the midwife replied firmly. "You're probably going to have several nights like this before you have a baby." Crestfallen, my husband went off to work and I went back to bed. I took several long naps during the day, while our nanny took our 2-year-old son to his playgroup and fed him lunch. My back ached and I had occasional mild contractions during the day, but nothing more.

"It won't be tonight," I thought on Wednesday evening. But just in case, I put the birthing pool together. It was sort of like a blue canvas tent on a five-foot-wide hexagonal frame, turned upside down. It filled to about 2 feet deep through a garden hose attached to a bathroom tap.

I went to bed at 10.30pm. Around midnight I found myself sitting up in bed in the middle of a contraction. I flopped back to sleep again between a few more contractions. Then I felt a trickle of water as though I'd wet the bed as my waters broke. I went to the bathroom for a pad and the contractions suddenly became very strong. For a while I sat on the sofa in our bedroom huffing and puffing. My husband kept on snoring. There didn't seem much point in waking him up—what could he do? It was still going to hurt. I went downstairs to try to distract myself. I guess contractions feel different for different people. I felt a stabbing pain in the small of my back that came in waves. One deep breath in, blow it away, another, another, soon it'll pass. Phew. It's gone. Then a rest before the next one begins. The day after my daughter was born, I told my brother, "It's like running a race" because my diaphragm felt bruised afterwards from breathing hard. But that's not quite correct. During a road race the pain is psychological as much as physical. You have to force yourself to keep running because if you don't, you will simply stop running and quit the race. But in labour, there's no quitting.

I could watch TV—would that help? I still hadn't looked at the instructional video that came with the birthing pool, so I put that on. Some stupid woman holding a baby was explaining in great detail how wonderful her water birth was. I switched her off and tried the end of *Singing in the Rain*, which we'd started watching a few days before. Couples in beautiful clothes waltzed to a brass band. Infuriating creatures. No, that wasn't what I needed.

The contractions were coming every few minutes. If I was sitting when one arrived, I stayed sitting and swayed back and forth, taking deep breaths and breathing out with a loud "Ooooh, ahhhhhh". Sitting seemed to lessen the pain along the bottom of my bump. If I was standing I paced to the end of the room and back, hollering the words to the *Battle Hymn of the Republic*. After a while, it didn't help to walk away from the pain. "This is no fun," I said to myself. "Remind me I said so next time I have the stupid idea that I want a baby. Nothing can possibly make this worthwhile!"

"Call me if you feel like you don't want to be by yourself any more," the midwife had said. I called her around 1.30am. "I don't like this any more." It was such a relief to do something besides pacing up and down the living room that I didn't even notice the next contraction. "If I can talk through a contraction, does that mean it's not that strong?" I asked.

"Well, usually that's right. But I can come out now if you want me to," she said, polite but unconvinced.

Oh dear. It's going to get much worse than this, I thought. "No, that's OK. Maybe I can survive a while longer."

I survived exactly 15 more minutes before I called her back. This time I was careful to make lots of convincing puffing noises during a contraction.

"I'll come right now," she said.

I can't remember what I did during the next 45 minutes. Knowing that help was on the way made the time fly. When I judged that she was about to arrive, I woke my husband up. His sleepy sense of decorum dictated that he should be fully dressed for her arrival. I went downstairs again to wait. I still remember the elation and relief I felt at the sound of the front gate creaking, then a clunk as she deposited her midwifery equipment on the doorstep.

The midwife kissed me when I opened the door. Another contraction arrived. "Breathe it out. You're doing great," she said, pressing her hands hard against the small of my back. My back felt less like it was going to fall off with her hands pressing against it. My husband came downstairs.

"We haven't filled the pool yet," I said. "Do you think we should?"

"I'll fill it," my husband offered.

"The hose attachment is in the top drawer in the bathroom, along with the spanner," I said. "It attaches to the shower." I had tried attaching the hose a few times myself to make sure it worked, but it hadn't occurred to me that someone else might need to know how to work it.

My husband was up on a stool in the bath when I made it upstairs. "The shower head won't come off," he said. "The spanner doesn't fit." "It fit when I tried it," I snapped, then grabbed for my back again as another contraction arrived.

"Shall I have a go?" The midwife climbed up on the stool, but couldn't make it work, either.

"Who do I have here? Two idiots?" I grumbled. "I don't believe this. I'm going to have to do it myself." I must have been in transition.

But five minutes later, he and the midwife attached the hose. "You can turn it on now," the midwife called from our bedroom. We could hear the water swishing through the hose. A minute later I heard myself exhale hard at the end of a contraction. I was hugging my husband. "That sounds weird," I thought to myself. "Am I pushing? I don't feel like I am. Am I supposed to be doing this?"

"That sounded like a pushing noise!" said the midwife, running in from the other room.

"I think I have to wee." I tried to sit on the toilet. "No, I think I have to poo."

"It sounds like you're pushing," she repeated. "We'd better check how far dilated you are."

It sounds like you're pushing, she repeated

After a few more contractions I made it to our bed, where the midwife felt my cervix. "You're fully dilated!" Seeing I didn't look pleased, she added: "That's good news!" I was thinking, "Oh no, now I'm going to have to push the baby out. What if I can't do it?"

"Would you like to get in the pool?" The midwife suggested. It was only half full but the water was rising quickly. The idea of moving or doing anything different sounded impossible, but I said I'd like to because I figured I was supposed to. I stepped out of my pyjamas and into the pool. The instant I felt the warm water over my ankles I felt better. The warm bath was instantly soothing, just as all the water birth brochures promised. It was even better than the firm pressure of someone's hands against my back. It was like being hugged all over.

The next contractions still hurt in the small of my back, but they were completely different. Before pushing begins it's a matter of passively enduring the pain. But when pushing starts, you feel like you're doing something. It felt sort of like throwing up—or should I say throwing down, because the involuntary hurling of the stomach muscles went down into my gut, not up into my throat. Pushing was scary, uncontrollable. I didn't know how long I could keep it up before my body ripped apart. "Just go with it," the midwife said. "You're doing great." She was kneeling next to the pool. I held onto the rim and crouched in the water. Before, looking straight into her eyes helped me remember that a contraction would end in another moment. Now I wasn't looking at her any more. I just held onto the rim of the pool and puked my stomach into my pelvis, then closed my eyes and took deep breaths when a break came. I was making heavy, pig-like exhaling noises. Soon after I got into the pool, our son woke up next door. "Mama!" My husband went in to sing him back to sleep. "No.... MAMA!" he protested.

Through the open door I tried to sing him a song between contractions, but quickly realised that he was just as happy listening to his favourite Papa story about the rabbit and the hedgehog.

I started to feel more pressure in my bowels. It sounds strange but the most pleasurable feeling was the hot sting of the perineum tearing as the baby's head crowned. The feeling of climax. The next push came immediately, and the baby's body squelched out into the water. And then everything stopped. No more pain. Instant peace. The midwife reached down and lifted the baby to the surface. Its face was a purple maroon, with slippery black hair matted down on its head. The baby looked very big to have just come out of my body. It breathed, then cried.

To avoid being disappointed if we ended up with two of the same, we'd convinced ourselves that we were having another son. "Now I get to check that it really is a boy," I thought. "The part I missed last time." I never got to see my first child as he was pulled out of my belly behind the screen on the operating table. The doctors took him away, suctioned his lungs, wrapped him up and presented him like a Christmas present, with nothing but a red, terrified and screaming face sticking out. He might as well have come from a factory. It took months before I was convinced he was my baby.

> He might as well have come from a factory. It took months before I was convinced he was my baby.

I lifted the baby's bottom toward the surface. I saw what looked like a scrotum. The rest of the crotch was blocked by the umbilical cord running from the navel, down between the legs and into the water. "Yep, a boy," I decided.

"You have a little girl," the midwife said. I took another look. Indeed, that was no penis I was looking at. Because of all the hormones in the mother's body, the baby's genitals come out all swollen. A daughter! I couldn't believe it. I put her to my breast, and she stopped crying. The midwife tiptoed to the door of our son's room.

"And then Rabbit said to Hedgehog..." my husband was saying.

"You have a little girl," she announced quietly.

My husband said later that he'd heard the baby crying but couldn't really believe that it had been born already.

> My husband said later that he'd heard the baby crying, but couldn't really believe that it had been born already

"Our client isn't going back to sleep," he reported to me. Our son appeared in the doorway. "Ooh!" he said, taking in the blue pool, the midwife, and his mother in the water. He padded up to the pool. "Baby!" he announced, looking at the slippery beet-red person in my arms.

"That's your sister," my husband said to him, his voice cracking. A few minutes later, sitting in the pool, I was on the phone to my mother and brother in Washington, DC.

My daughter and I sat in the water and breastfed for nearly an hour until the cord stopped pulsing. The midwife clamped the cord next to the baby's navel, then cut through the tough, horny tube. A moment later, the placenta slid out like a big jellyfish.

"Is it true that eating a piece of placenta helps the uterus contract?"

"Yes, though I only know two people who've actually tried it."

> "I only know two people who've actually tried it"

"I did last time, but it was probably pointless because it was after I came back from the hospital. And it must have been filled with epidural drugs and other awful chemicals. I ate a bit raw."

"What did you do with the rest of it? Bury it in the garden?"

"Um, no. I fried it up with onions and ate the whole thing."

"Oh," she said politely. We examined the placenta to make sure no part had been left in the uterus. She pulled off a small, meaty piece. "This is probably enough to help your uterus contract." It was like eating warm, raw liver.

My husband and son came back from cooking up a pot of porridge. I climbed out of the pool carrying my newborn daughter. We all watched as the midwife weighed her in a sling: 8lb 6oz—nearly a pound over her brother's birth weight. Then the midwife sewed me up. My perineum had a fairly long but shallow tear from the bottom of the vagina toward the anus, which the midwife said looked like it wasn't sitting together tidily and might heal in an uncomfortable way if it wasn't sewn up. She injected a surface anaesthetic, the only drug which appears in my birth notes, then put in four stitches. It was nearly 7.00am when we finished our porridge. I can't remember now who was holding the baby. All I can remember is how famished I was. I was watching the clock. I couldn't wait until the nanny arrived so I could show off my good work. My husband had paged her to come at 8.00am, an hour earlier than usual. When I heard her key in the lock, I wanted to leap down the stairs with the baby in my arms. "But she'll tell me to go right back to bed," I thought. I suddenly realised I was exhausted.

I was on such a high that day, I even briefly went out. We invited a few friends over in the evening to celebrate with a glass of champagne. Afterwards, I slightly regretted disturbing our baby by inviting other people into her new home. I am ashamed to confess that in the photos of her birthday party she is screaming her head off as she's passed around. By the time I descended from Cloud 9 enough to feel like resting, the baby had got over her initial post-birth calm and wanted to breastfeed frequently. I should have slept when she slept! (Mental note: Stay in bed next time and keep visitors away.)

During the day my daughter was born, I could still remember exactly what the sickening wave of a contraction felt like. By the next morning I wasn't sure any more. Did it really hurt that much?

Some days I feel weepy and nostalgic. I'd like to be back in the blue plastic pool, pushing my daughter—my daughter!—into the world. She's three weeks old now. Some days I miss being pregnant. How strange from one moment to the next to change from a beautiful, rotund, mum-to-be into a tired, empty-bellied mother. Now that life has gone back to normal, I wish I could be pregnant and special again. I miss the feeling of somebody's feet kicking inside me. But then I reach out my hand to touch our daughter's soft, downy head and I remember how I pushed her out into the world. Life won't ever go back to 'normal'… our daughter is here for keeps.

Post scriptum by Nina:

Our third child was born after a similar five hours of established labour, five and a half years later. The contractions in this labour felt much more painful than in the second one. Boy, did it hurt! (They do say third births are sometimes tougher. Or maybe I noticed the pain more. I was expecting it to be a piece of cake!) This time, I did take it easy and let people wait on me. Like her big sister, the new one was calm and happy after the birth, and so were her older brother and sister.

I would gladly re-live the births of either of my daughters. There is nothing more intensely satisfying than labouring and birthing a baby. I wish I could do it again a dozen times more. It's bringing them up that's hard work!

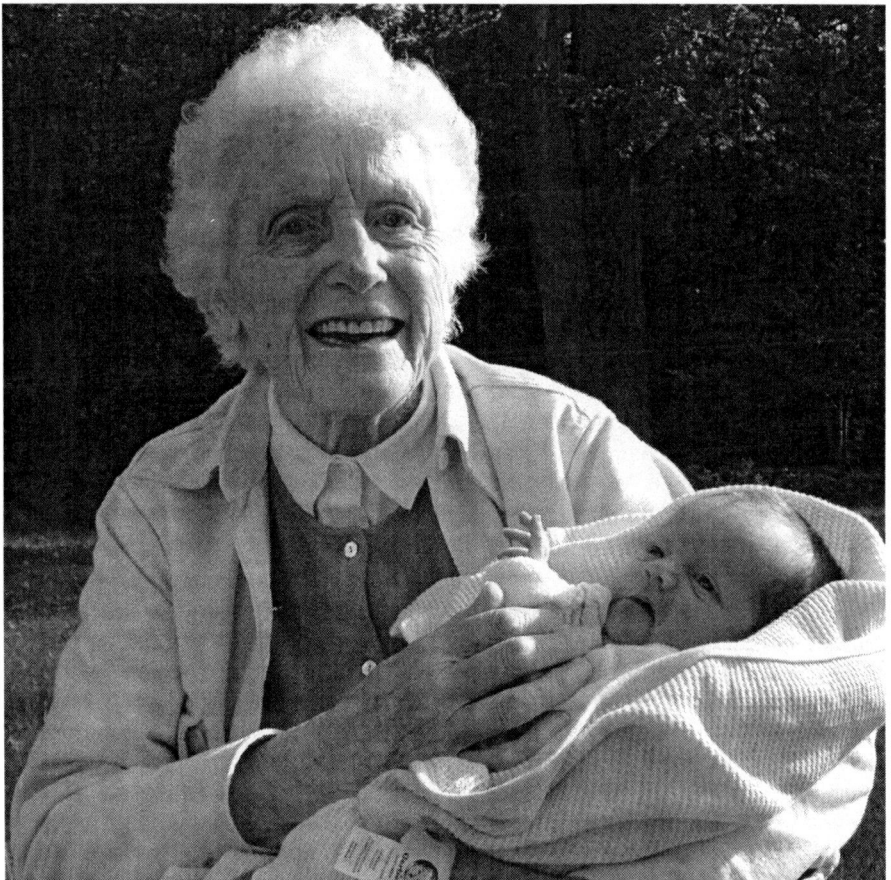

Nina's second baby, Sophia, with her great-grandmother Celina Robbins, who was also born at home—in 1916. The two intervening generations were born in hospital, Eliza in 'twilight sleep' in 1940 and Nina in an unmedicated 'natural' hospital birth in 1967.

Confronting fears

Maria Shanahan

I was very frightened about my ability to give birth properly, and questioned all my ideas about home and water birth. I called the Active Birth Centre in London and explained my experiences at the hospital when I had my first baby, Fiohann. I asked if there was anyone I could talk it through with. They gave me a few names, and then suggested Michel Odent. I couldn't believe that I actually had my revered Michel Odent's phone number.

Before I could think about it, I forced myself to phone him. I explained to him what had happened and although, understandably, he wasn't prepared to comment on the hospital treatment, he did explain that not many midwives had experience of water births and could panic, thinking the baby would drown. I told him it was a dream of mine that he would deliver our baby and, after hearing when the conception date was, he found that it did fit in with his schedule of international conferences and that, yes, he would. I had to pinch myself!

He came around to meet us and I cannot describe what a gentle, intuitive and passionate man he is. He filled me with a quiet confidence and reassurance and was so different to our doctor, who had originally told me that if I wanted a home birth I would have to find another doctor. Another difference was that he had absolutely no problem with calculating the due date from the conception date: it was a simple nine months later. The community midwife could not cope with anything more than the date of my last period, which I did not know exactly, since I never paid any attention to my cycle. Her date was two weeks before Michel's estimate. The pregnancy went well in that I was fit and healthy, but my partner and I started to have problems and when I was six months pregnant he left home for a month. I felt desperately insecure and cried through most of my pregnancy. Another pregnancy filled with grief, but so different to the first. We went on holiday and decided to try again.

I hired the birthing pool two days before the earliest due date and waited. The midwife got increasingly agitated and by 21 July was telling me that I would be causing the fetus brain damage because my placenta was past its sell-by date. Michel calmed her by telling her it was due on the 26th, which she could not comprehend. Sure enough, on the 25th, which happily was a Saturday, I went into labour. I called Michel and he promised to be over in a couple of hours. We filled the pool, put the low music on and had candles ready, and I tried to relax, but found it difficult because of my doubts in myself. Michel arrived and asked me how I was, felt my tummy, and said he would go to sleep in the next room as I had a few hours to go yet. My partner went to sleep in our bed and I spent most of the night sitting on the loo having contractions. It felt the most comfortable place to be, looking at the stars through the bathroom roof window and going back to bed trying to doze before the next contraction.

Early next morning, things started hotting up and I decided to get into the birthing pool to ease the pains. It did ease them immediately and, as soon as he heard the change in my noises, Michel got up and came in. He can tell where a woman is in her labour by the noises she makes and just that small change had indicated to him a change in me. I told him I didn't know what to do and asked him what I should be doing. So different from my first birth... he told me just to listen to my body, just as I had done in the first. I yelled that I didn't know what it was saying, and was very fearful. How different to the first time, with my confidence now in tatters. He calmly created an environment where I would have to listen to myself, by leaving me alone and getting my partner to go and have some breakfast. Our Brazilian au pair was beside herself that I could be moaning and wailing alone with no doctor and took it into her own hands to go and tell Michel in no uncertain terms to go in to me and induce me! In Brazil, apparently, over 40% of women have caesarean sections because it keeps their passages honeymoon fresh! He handled her sweetly and reassured her. [Actually, the rate is now more like 90% in cities!]

Things really got going at about 8.30am. I was gnawing on the side of the birthing pool, thinking about the benefits of knives and drugs, half hoping that she wouldn't come out at all, would go back and stay safe inside me.

But that doesn't happen, and finally I got that huge push urge, when all you can do is that colossal push and your whole body is intent on turning itself inside out.

It did know after all what to do, I just had to get my doubts out of the way. Her head came out in the water, just like Fiohann—my son. Michel reached down and checked the umbilical cord was not in the way and then said that because she was so big we needed gravity to help us. With her head still between my legs, he lifted my legs and my partner lifted my torso out of the pool. I hung from his arms with Michel ready to catch her.

Two more big pushes and out she slid, our beautiful girl.

I flopped to the floor and Michel gave her to me immediately. I held her close and within a few minutes she was nuzzling at my breast ready to suckle, still attached to the umbilical cord.

Michel was delighted at the perfection of it but said that before she settled into it he would tie off her cord with string rather than the metal clamps because it was more comfortable for the baby. I lay on our bed with our wonderful baby and as she suckled I realised that it would have been no different for Fiohann. If only.

Michel left me to deliver Eowyn's placenta naturally, which came easily shortly afterwards. What I hadn't expected was the sharper pains as my uterus contracted back again, but apparently this is a normal feature of a second childbirth.

Michel wrote to our doctor to inform him of the birth and our baby's 'top' scores, knowing that we would be left undisturbed until Monday. Once again, I had no tears and was perfectly fit. The day following Eowyn's birth we had a celebration barbecue and I walked around Tesco's shopping for it, feeling so proud and happy, as if everyone must be able to tell that I had just had a baby! Michel came with his son and was thrilled to see us so clearly well and happy. It was perfect.

Our doctor and his doctor wife arrived Monday morning, demanding to know how long the baby sucked on each breast and making appointments for paediatricians to see her. I had no idea how long on each breast and I declined the paediatrician offer, which they seemed a bit put out about.

Finally they left, leaving the midwives and health visitors to do their checks, etc and eventually we were left in peace again.

As I write this, Eowyn is now a very fit and healthy 4-year-old.

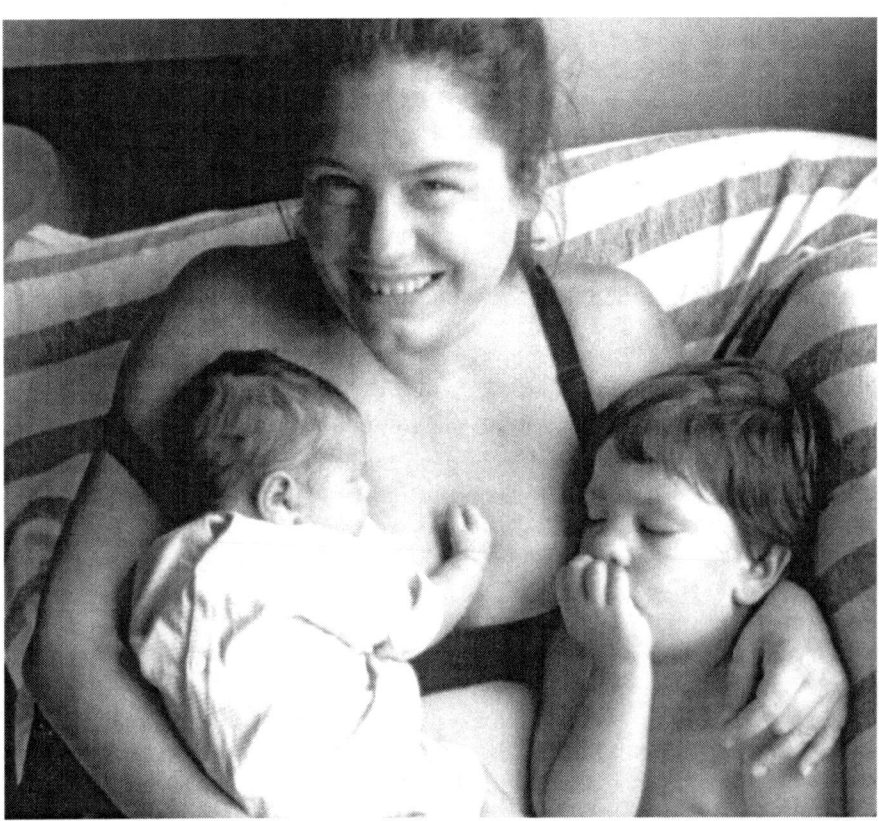

Maria with Eowyn and Fiohann when they were little

Homebirth healing

Anon

My first baby was a planned hospital birth. I expected to just turn up in labour, have the baby and come home. I didn't really take on board the 'cascade of intervention' which can and does happen in hospitals to upset the natural balance of a labour that is going well. After a traumatic forceps delivery the consultant was clearly in a hurry to get the placenta out and pulled vigorously on the cord—this is not only bad practice, as controlled cord traction should be used, but is dangerous and possibly negligent. I lost 1500ml of blood within seconds, fainted and when I came round needed a blood transfusion.

> I expected to just turn up in labour, have the baby and come home. I didn't really take on board the 'cascade of intervention' which can and does happen.

My next baby was a planned home birth—I could not imagine going to hospital and going through the same thing. I booked with community midwives who are generally supportive of home birth but when my history of a PPH [postpartum haemorrhage] was revealed (by me, voluntarily) I was told that a homebirth would be out of the question. I was made to feel that my body was at fault for pouring out a life-threatening amount of blood after giving birth. The truth, however, was that mismanagement had caused the heavy blood loss.

I soon booked with independent midwives, who had the confidence in my body which I had, and gave birth to a second daughter at home in under three hours. This was a totally straightforward birth with no time for the TENS, birthing pool or gas and air, which I had planned. I stood up for delivery, supported by my partner and pushed the baby out myself, the midwife 'catching' her well. I had no injection to speed up the placenta and control the blood loss as it was just not necessary and this third stage was completed in about 20 minutes.

I was on such a high for ages—I felt empowered and I had re-gained the confidence in my own body which my first birth had taken away. I don't feel that I did anything either 'brave' or 'dangerous' by giving birth at home. I felt very safe and it was right for me.

> I was on such a high for ages—I felt empowered and I had re-gained the confidence in my own body, which my first birth had taken away. I don't feel that I did anything either 'brave' or 'dangerous' by giving birth at home. I felt very safe and it was right for me.

Testing the limits of possibility...

Sometimes couples choose to do things a little differently. Sometimes circumstances *force* them to proceed differently. Considering a few of these cases can be inspirational and can even sometimes prompt us to improve things, even when we give birth in more conventional ways, particularly when we personally have particular problems to overcome, which seem insuperable.

In the first account we meet one of the growing number of women who are choosing to give birth without the assistance of medical personnel. These women—who are usually highly educated women (in particular in the USA and Russia)—are proving that modern woman still has the inborn ability to birth her babies, without instruction or support from caregivers. Laura Shanley, who has birthed all of her four children 'unassisted' (at least by the medical profession)—and who contributed the following story—suggests that *every* woman (modern or primitive) has the inborn ability to give birth, provided any ingrained fear, guilt or shame can be overcome. She helped overcome her own negative feelings through what she calls 'belief suggestions'; in other words, she repeatedly 'thought' statements which reflected what she wanted to believe, either on an ongoing basis or at key moments. Her husband completely supports this approach. He also believes that natural, undisturbed, home-based birthing is best because he says traumatic childbirth diminishes the mother-child relationship, starts a person off on a rocky start and is ultimately to blame for many of society's ills.

Of course, the practice of intentionally giving birth without medical assistance (freebirth) is highly controversial, even though its safety record is good. Laura has worked to publicise the advantages of 'going it alone' through her website www.unassistedchildbirth.com, her book *Unassisted Childbirth* and her film *A Clear Road to Birth*. Whatever our personal position on this issue, it is truly remarkable to consider how straightforward a birth can be—in this case an unexpected footling breech—when a female body and her baby are left to labour entirely without disturbance and when both mother and baby experience birth without fear.

In the second account, the woman had no choice but to give birth alone... and in the two accounts after that we read about women who gave birth in unusual circumstances. One woman, who was ill with multiple sclerosis, got herself psyched up to experiencing pain through systematic preparation. The other one had to overcome enormous psychological blocks which had developed as a result of being sexually abused as a child. In the last account, we read about a woman who tested the limits of possibility by daring to find out what would happen if she *didn't* cut the baby's umbilical cord after the birth.

Whether or not you relate to any of these situations and decisions, reading about them could certainly prompt decisions which are right for you personally.

Going it alone

Laura Shanley

A year and a half after giving birth to my first son John, I realised I was pregnant with Willie. Once again, I had a very healthy pregnancy. I never experienced morning sickness or had any of the other so-called 'symptoms' of pregnancy (which I believe are often fear-induced). I decided I would give birth on my hands and knees because that had worked so well with John, but in a dream I was shown otherwise. In the dream, I was watching a woman giving birth standing up. She was straddling a little plastic baby bathtub and catching the baby herself. As I watched her, I heard another woman very gently say to me, "Tell her to remember not to do too much." I understood what the woman was saying and the peaceful feeling of the dream stayed with me for the remainder of my pregnancy. I want to say at this point that I don't follow every dream I have, but this dream was different. It seemed to be coming from the deepest part of my being. And so, I decided to follow it faithfully—I would catch my baby myself as I stood over my little bathtub, and I would move out of the way and essentially do nothing to interfere with the process.

On the morning of 17 August, I began to feel contractions. David and I made love and I remember feeling an orgasm followed immediately by a contraction. The rhythmic contracting of my uterus during the orgasm felt almost identical to that of the contraction. They seemed to have the same pattern, although I must admit the orgasm felt better! A few minutes later, I was walking across the room when my waters broke. I took out my little bathtub and stood over it as I had been shown in the dream. At that point I couldn't feel the contractions but I knew I was having them because when I put my hand inside my vagina I could feel my pelvic muscles rhythmically contracting around it. A few minutes later a foot appeared between my legs. I wasn't expecting a breech birth, although a friend of mine told me during my pregnancy that he had dreamt he saw the baby inside me standing right-side-up.

David and I said 'belief suggestions' that everything would be all right and then we patiently waited for Willie to be born. Little by little his foot got lower and soon his other foot popped out. When I felt the time was right I gave one push and gently pulled him out by the feet. David and John had been in the other room but walked in just as Willie emerged. David yelled excitedly, "You did it!" and Willie immediately began to nurse. Incidentally, 12 years later I read that Michel Odent says that for a breech delivery a woman should always be in a 'standing squat' or 'upright' position and an attendant should do absolutely nothing to interfere, if at all possible. This was the message of the dream.

Soon after the birth I dreamt that Willie was speaking to me. He told me that part of the reason his birth had been so fast and easy—he was born two hours after the first contraction—was that he hadn't been afraid either. Babies are always picking up on our beliefs, both before and after birth, so a fearless mother means a fearless baby.

Today, Willie is a happy and fearless 22-year-old!

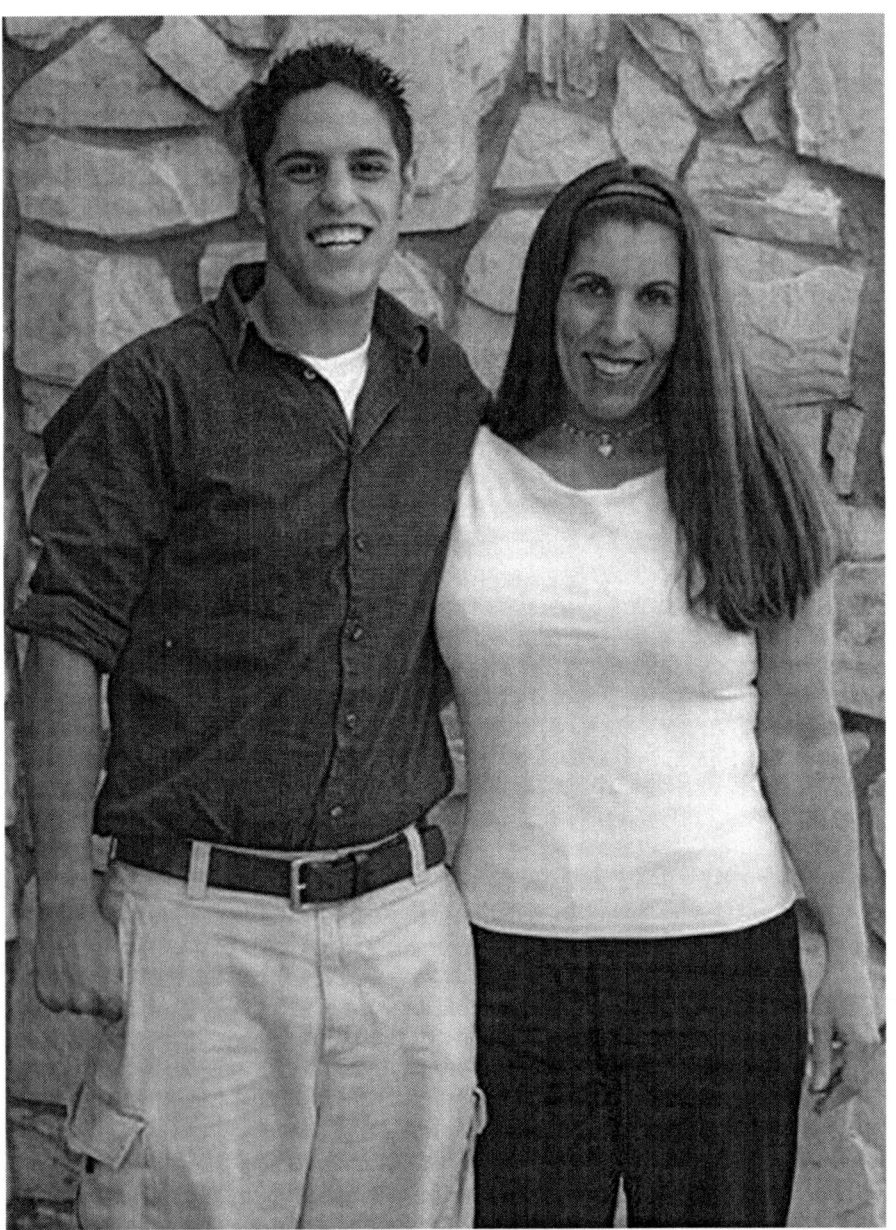

Willie and Laura—summer 2002

Being taken by surprise

Tanya Kudryashova

I was 34 when my husband and I decided to have a second child. We were much more careful about everything than with the first. Two years before I conceived, my husband entirely gave up alcohol—even wine and beer—because he wanted to have a healthy baby. I went to my obstetrician for a check-up and tried to stay healthy too.

I went for a check-up and tried to stay healthy too

When we discovered the baby was on the way, I started collecting information about the best way to go about things. I found out about a number of childbirth preparation schools and signed up for a course with a midwife and teacher at a local 'family centre'. The atmosphere there was so wonderful. There was an almost magical warmth in the classes. At the end of each class I left feeling full of love for the entire world. One of the most important things the teacher did, I think, was prepare the mother to love her baby. I mean, of course you love your baby, that's natural. But she made you view the whole process as a joint effort, as something special. She made me think about helping the baby, not just helping myself. I began to want the birth to go well for the baby, too.

Usually women think of the future birth as a trial not only for them, but for the child, too. Most women think about themselves and getting through the birth—whether to have painkillers or not, whether they might end up with a caesarean or not. This teacher helped us to see that the birth is a powerful and challenging experience for the child too.

When we found out we were having twins, I expected I would have the babies in hospital. But then I saw a video about a woman who had twins at home, in a birthing pool. I certainly didn't expect to have a home birth but the more I learnt, the more I found out it would be best for both me and the babies. I wanted them to be able to be with me from their first minutes. I so much wanted their first moments after birth to be good and happy for them. So I started planning a home birth.

I visited a lot of birth centres. A month before they were born, I did a second scan. My doctor saw that they were both head-down, with no sign of the cords around their necks, with a fairly good weight and no visible pathology. So everything seemed fine. On the other hand, during the last month I found it very difficult to walk because of the pressure of their heads in my pelvis. Maybe because I have a narrow pelvis, I felt shooting pains in my legs every time I stood up. So the last month or even two months I spent nearly all my time in bed.

The more I learnt, the more I found out it would be best

My obstetrician told me that since it was twins they might be born prematurely, so we thought about what to do. But I knew that if I went to hospital, most likely the babies would be taken to the special care nursery at first. I suddenly began to feel very confident that I should try to have them at home. I made plans with my midwife. The babies came three weeks early.

Sometime around midnight, or maybe a bit after, my waters broke. I began to feel mild contractions. I called the midwife and she asked me to check how far dilated I was. At around 4.00am, my husband, who had got the car ready, went to pick up the midwife. The contractions were becoming stronger and more frequent. I coped with the pain using the natural methods we learned in the birth classes: breathing, moving around, massage. My mother started cleaning the bath and getting some sea salt to put in the water. [Russian birth classes recommend adding sea salt to the water in a birthing pool or bath. The iodine in the sea salt is thought to kill germs; the salt is thought to be healthy for the baby to be born into]. My older son, who was 9 at the time, was home too, but he was very nervous. He went into the other room and closed the door. We didn't bother him.

The labour progressed very quickly and at a certain point I realised that I was about to give birth alone, without my midwife. I felt not so much panic but utter loneliness, realising that I was going to have to give birth on my own. And then I summoned my strength. I realised "Everything is going to be OK." I pulled myself together and began to think about what I needed to do. Thanks to everything I had learnt in the birth class, I knew I would find the strength in myself.

I started feeling that I had to push. My mother hadn't even had time to get the bath ready or fill it. So I went over and lay down on the bed. I lay on my back because it felt more comfortable. It was purely an instinctive thing. I didn't think what I should do or what I needed. Nature dictated how I should behave. My mother was right there. The first head appeared. I told my mother: "Don't touch the baby. Wait until the shoulders are born. Then you can pull the baby out." The obstetrician had told me from the scan that we were having two boys. My mother, who is a paediatrician, caught the first baby. She put him on my tummy. I don't remember it but she tells me that she saw him crawl up my chest to find the breast. He latched on and began to breastfeed. We didn't clean him off, as we had been told in the birth classes, but just let the amniotic fluid soak in. Soon his skin turned pink and glowing.

About 20 minutes later, the second birth began. It was probably harder for the first one since he had to open the path, so to speak. The second one came out very quickly. The contractions were quite strong and painful. I've heard of women giving birth with no pain, but it certainly wasn't like that for me. My mother put the second baby on my tummy. I wasn't looking at the baby carefully, I was just concentrating on her beginning. "I don't think it's a boy!" my mother said. My daughter had trouble breathing at first and sucking wasn't easy for her. The midwife arrived and looked at the babies. She said we must cut the cord for the girl right away. About three hours later, my husband cut our son's cord himself. He was so proud!

The babies were born with two placentas; each child had had its own sac. The midwife checked the condition of the placentas. We weighed the babies with one of those spring scales you use for weighing vegetables at the market. Liza weighed 6lb 13oz (3.1kg), Dmitry weighed 6lb 7oz (2.9kg). Of course, it wasn't 100% accurate, but pretty close. Later that week, my husband bought some electronic weighing scales. By that point their weight had stabilised, and they began gaining steadily. From the very first day, we bathed them daily and did baby massage with them.

During the first three weeks, the babies stayed with me all the time. I held them on my chest to keep them warm. I was very weak at first. I lost 5kg relative to my weight before the birth, 55 kg. I gained about 15 kg during the pregnancy. Once a week, I followed the fasting diet recommended in the birth classes: for breakfast, only juices and fresh salads, then juices only for the rest of the day. Because of the inspiring birth preparation classes, I found I didn't even feel like eating sweets. You understand that healthy food is best and want to eat those things. I think I needed this kind of regimen to get to full term. It's not necessary to gain masses of weight. With a smaller weight gain, the child still takes what it needs. It's better to have natural foods than to take extra, artificial vitamins.

I breastfed exclusively for five or six months—no juices or water, just breast-milk. They breastfed until about a year and three months. We did lots of exercises with them and baby massage and took long walks in the fresh air. In the early days I was nothing but a milk machine! I hardly had time for anything else. I would just get one fed, when it'd be time to feed the other one again. Now they are 3 years, 2 months old and weigh 2st 4lb (15kg).

Adjusting to pain

Gemma Shepherd

When my first baby Kizzy was born in hospital I felt very empowered by the birth. I had used no drugs of any sort and had no interventions, yet I couldn't imagine wanting to repeat it. "How does anyone ever have more than one baby?" I asked my mum the next day.

However, a year or so later a friend at a La Leche League meeting about birth recommended *Spiritual Midwifery* by Ina May Gaskin. The book is full of stories about peaceful, joyful home births. It was a complete revelation to me that birth could be totally painfree and enjoyable. I thought a lot about changing my view of pain and began to see contractions as 'rushes of energy'. I learned to relax my body and to think of pain as 'an interesting sensation that I needed to concentrate on'.

In the book it is often said that if the mouth is 'soft' (i.e. relaxed), then the pelvic floor area will be too. I practised this by blowing out through my mouth with very relaxed lips when I went to the toilet. I also tried not to tense up when I experienced any sort of pain. For instance, if I stubbed my toe I would relax myself and the pain lessened much more quickly than normally. I was able to combine Ina May Gaskin's theories about pain with Michel Odent's writings about a woman's instinctive understanding of what positions to adopt during labour and birth. (After all, most—if not all?—of the women in *Spiritual Midwifery* had given birth in bed, on their backs or semi-reclined.)

I had a sort of practice run at birth when I had a miscarriage when Kizzy was 20 months old. After two weeks of spotting blood, a mini-labour began when I was 12 weeks pregnant. I knew the baby had died because I had stopped feeling pregnant around the time the bleeding had started. (I had also had a scan where they 'informed' me there was no heartbeat, as if I didn't know what was going on in my body.) I relaxed through the miscarriage and it was painless. I could sense that the feelings would have been painful, much like strong period cramps, if I had been tense. I felt elated when it was over, as if I had really achieved something by not feeling any pain. I wasn't ready for another baby yet and felt that the miscarriage had been for the best. (I had another scan afterwards where they 'let me know' that my uterus was now empty!)

My next pregnancy was planned and the baby was due when Kizzy was 3½. By this time we had moved from London, where the maternity care was very impersonal, to a small, fairly isolated town. The local hospital has a midwife-run maternity unit and the midwives are friendly, relaxed and have plenty of time to chat. Even so, I knew I would have a home birth this time. I planned a water birth and hired a pool as (even though I was much more confident that I could cope with the contractions) I still felt that a pool would provide some pain relief if I needed it, and the calm, enveloping warmth of the water was appealing.

My team of four midwives seemed keen on the water birth and had special training sessions at another hospital to prepare them. None had delivered a baby in water before and I think they had little experience of home birth. By the end of my pregnancy I felt fully prepared for the birthing to come.

Dora was born at home on a beautiful sunny morning in June 2000. The labour was fairly quick. My waters broke at midnight and I tried to sleep, but was too excited. I had a long bath instead and meditated and visualised my womb opening up to let my baby out. I managed some sleep, but by 4 o'clock the contractions were coming regularly. I felt very peaceful and safe as I pottered around the silent, sleeping house, tidying and arranging things for the midwives. When a contraction came, I would lean on a piece of furniture or the kitchen side and sway gently, breathing slowly out through my mouth.

I meditated and visualised my womb opening up

Each contraction was like an exciting journey—enjoyable in itself, but also promising even better to come. I felt the love of friends and family like a warm glow, especially when I was looking at various photos around the house. Even though I was alone physically, I knew there were many people with me in spirit. I often smiled and laughed during contractions and when one was over I waited eagerly for the next.

Jim, my husband, called the midwife at about 7 o'clock, when I felt things were progressing, then began to fill the pool. The midwife arrived and checked me just before 8.00am—I was 3cm dilated. This surprised me as I thought I was further along, but as things turned out maybe I was.

After a few more contractions things began to intensify. I remember moaning 'Woaah' as the feelings suddenly became much stronger. There was still no pain, though I had to work much harder to stay relaxed enough. (I realised after that this was probably transition.) I decided to get into the pool now, thinking I might not be able to cope if things got any stronger. The water felt wonderful, like a big, warm hug. I had two more contractions, then with the next—out of the blue—I had an overwhelming urge to push. The midwife, who was waiting for the other midwife to arrive, shouted "No!" when I told her. I understood then that she was scared to be on her own. I didn't let her fear affect me but when I pushed during that contraction some diarrhoea came out. The midwife insisted I leave the pool as she thought it was too contaminated to give birth in.

Although I had expected to want to squat to give birth, my body knew that it needed to stand and my knees straightened up automatically. I leaned on the side of the pool. During the first push I had felt the baby move down rapidly. With the next, the head crowned and I reached down to touch Dora's soft hair. I had to slow myself down at this stage to be sure I didn't push too hard. I stopped pushing mid-contraction and breathed slowly. I was aware of the beauty of the sunny, blue sky outside and the wonderment of the moment. I felt a strong connection with all of nature. Then the final contraction, and the head was born. I looked down and clearly recall how surreal it seemed to see her head between my legs. I reminded myself to go slowly and within a few seconds her whole body slid gently out.

I held her and she cried with her eyes tight shut for several minutes—it was probably very bright for her. Dora was born at 9.18am, less than an hour and a half since I was examined at 3cm dilated. Kizzy and Jim came into the room, amazed to see a baby. They had been making breakfast in the kitchen when Kizzy said she could hear a baby crying. Jim wasn't sure at first because he thought there was still some way to go!

Dora suckled for the first time and the placenta was delivered a few minutes later. Unfortunately, the midwife pulled on the cord as the placenta was coming out. This was totally unnecessary, felt quite uncomfortable to me and could have created problems.

Dora's birth was serene and peaceful, full of joy and love—something to be cherished. I was on such a high to have achieved my dream of a totally painfree birth and to have my beautiful baby girl in my arms. The only thing to mar the experience was the midwives' interference, however minor. Luckily, I was strong and aware of my body to the extent that I was able to ignore the negative aspects of the midwifery 'care' and still feel I had had the best experience of my life. I was eager to give birth again!

Facing deep-down memories

Beth Dubois

I have been enthralled by stories of empowering births since my college years, when I made the acquaintance of several home birth midwives. However, I was disappointed by the so-called natural childbirth I witnessed during my education as a nurse, when I was required to attend several hospital births. The midwives were zealously cheering "Push! Push! I want to see this baby! Push!" No one was encouraging the woman to follow what her body and baby were doing naturally. It seemed the woman was expected to birth her baby for the midwives rather than to be present in her own experience.

When I became pregnant, I knew I wanted something different. I wanted to feel safe and comfortable so that I could open and allow my baby to be born. In addition, I am a survivor of childhood sexual abuse and I knew that the 'wrong' environment could trigger flashbacks and definitely impede the birthing process, possibly even creating further emotional trauma. On the other hand, I hoped that an empowering birth experience could promote healing at a very deep level. In a way my background as a survivor was a gift, as it led me on an intensive inner and outer quest for a healing pregnancy and birth. As I can see now, the process of undergoing the journey, in itself, was healing.

My husband and I spent endless hours reading and discussing aspects of antenatal care and birthing. We interviewed five home birth midwives and two midwifery group practices. We changed caregivers three times, wavered for months when trying to decide between a home birth, birth centre birth and hospital birth. Finally, we decided we felt most comfortable with a planned home birth, with a midwifery practice as our back-up, should a hospital birth become necessary. We took a great childbirth class based on the book *Birthing from Within* by Pam England and Rob Horowitz, which prepared us for the birth in a very experiential way. In the class, we practised pain-coping techniques—while holding ice cubes to simulate the pain of contractions!—discussed and faced fears, did birth artwork, and watched videos of women labouring and birthing in very non-interventionist settings.

I delighted in the physical closeness I had with my baby during my last few months of pregnancy. I loved to feel him move and to touch and massage his various parts. In fact, even when I was 40 weeks pregnant I felt very comfortable with my baby inside me; I didn't experience the feeling of 'wanting this baby out' or 'wanting to get my body back' that many women describe. And then 41 weeks came and went. As comfortable and wonderful as it was having him so close, I also longed to meet this new person and become a mother. Actually, there was also a sense of urgency because we were due to move to another area a fortnight later! During this period of waiting (and trying many techniques to induce labour) I had plenty of time to worry about various things, mostly related to the birth and the move. At a certain point, my anxieties began to centre on breastfeeding. As a nurse, I was well versed in the benefits of breastfeeding and had a lot of 'book knowledge' on the subject; I was certain that I wanted to breastfeed. I was extremely concerned, however, that I would not be able to comfortably maintain the constant physical closeness and literally the suckling that breastfeeding would require. I was concerned that breastfeeding would trigger memories of my childhood abuse.

My midwives knew about the sexual abuse and we had discussed it in terms of the birth, but I had felt ashamed and afraid to bring up the topic of how my background might affect breastfeeding. As is common with abuse survivors, I carried the shame of the abuse. I felt I was the only one who had ever faced these issues and also, illogically, that admitting their existence might 'jinx' the breastfeeding. I was especially distraught because I believed from the core of my being that I would be failing my child and myself in a very profound way if I were not able to breastfeed.

Eventually, at 41 weeks and still counting, I knew I needed help! I could find no information about survivors of sexual abuse and breastfeeding in any of the literature. I took a courageous step and arranged for a meeting with a lactation consultant who came highly recommended. She listened to my fears and reflections and gave me a lot of reassurance. She said that I had a great chance of successfully breastfeeding. Women who have been sexually abused sometimes have trouble tolerating the physical closeness breastfeeding requires, as was my fear for myself, but different women behave differently when faced with new motherhood as a survivor of abuse. Some lose confidence in their bodies and worry that they will not be capable of producing enough milk. For others, the physical sensations involved with breastfeeding may remind them of the abuse they suffered, which was also something I was concerned about.

After speaking to the lactation consultant, I felt so much freer... my 'secret' was out. I then felt comfortable discussing the issues with my midwives—it turned out they were not at all surprised and had faced these same issues with other women before. I felt so relieved. Both my shame and fear decreased.

Our home birth midwife, Ann, said that many women with abuse backgrounds and/or who do not feel comfortable with nipple stimulation by their partner have no problem when they breastfeed a baby. She said that the hormones released by breastfeeding make women able to tolerate and even enjoy the close contact with their babies. Our midwife, Valerie, told me that it was the love that mattered in feeding the baby, whether from breast or bottle. She said I should try to breastfeed and see what happened. Of course, I still desperately wanted to be able to breastfeed, but I felt less pressure after hearing her words.

At Valerie's suggestion, I took some time to write about my fears and realised that breastfeeding a baby really would be different from the abusive situation I was in as a child. My baby, tiny and in need of food, warmth, and love, would be totally different from the adult who had abused me. And as a breastfeeding mother, I would be in a totally different position than the one I was in as a child suffering the abuse. Instead of being a small child overpowered by someone huge and terrifying, I would be a grown woman responding very naturally to my baby's needs. These insights gave me hope that I would succeed at breastfeeding.

I also prayed that I would be able to breastfeed. To me, being able to successfully breastfeed seemed like a quantum leap. It seemed like it truly would be nothing short of a miracle. I didn't have time to do more therapy, more healing, because my baby would be here any day... I needed grace! So I prayed that somehow, just somehow, I would be able to successfully breastfeed.

As the days wore on I continued to be anxious that our baby was not yet born. Our move date was rapidly approaching and, to make things worse, I knew that at two weeks after our due date the policy of both our home birth midwife and midwifery practice was for us to have our birth in the hospital. 'Nesting' was difficult, to say the least!

Suddenly at 13 days after our due date, I had a surprising inner shift and felt that the right thing for me to do was go to the hospital and try a very gentle labour induction—prostaglandin gel on my cervix (which is not the same as Cytotec, incidentally). My husband and I spoke to our midwives, who agreed with our plan. It was in fact Valerie who was the midwife on call. From our earlier conversations, I knew that she was very experienced in working with women with sexual abuse backgrounds. I also knew she recognised and appreciated the inner work I had done and that she welcomed the opportunity to attend our birth. I felt safe with the thought of being in Valerie's care. She said: "We'll make it just like a home birth. Come at 7.30 or 8.00pm and decorate your room. We can start the induction after that." My husband and I spent the day grieving that we weren't having the home birth we had hoped for and packing up everything we wanted to have with us.

We were welcomed warmly by the midwives. Valerie had even 'reserved' a specific room for us which had a huge jacuzzi tub. Our home birth midwife, Ann, met us at the hospital, which gave me a strong sense of protection. When we saw Valerie and I told her that we didn't want to be there, that we wanted a home birth, she said: "OK. Then go home." But I was clear I did want to try to have my baby right then, so we stayed. However, knowing that no one was insisting on my being at the hospital kept me feeling in control (which was clearly Valerie's intention). We decorated our room a bit. Then Valerie inserted the prostaglandin gel and explained it was a 12-hour slow release. I would need to have fetal monitoring continuously for two hours (to make sure it wasn't releasing too quickly) and then we could go to sleep and see if anything happened in the morning. We never did go to sleep... To my great delight, within two hours I was having strong regular contractions. After the monitor was unhooked, Joel (my husband) and I walked up and down the halls, up and down the stairs, talking and laughing. I was so excited to finally be having regular contractions. I was even happy about the pain.

Wanting to just be alone with Joel, I asked him to ask Ann to leave, that we would call her when labour really got underway (as we were still under the impression that nothing much would happen until the morning). As soon as Ann left, I felt the intensity of the contractions increase. I got in the jacuzzi tub. Lying there in the dark, warm water and listening to the whirring of the jets, I felt like I myself was in the womb. As the contractions got stronger my focus became completely inward.

I remembered a slogan from *Birthing from Within*: 'Relax, breathe, do nothing extra'. I chanted "Om" during the contractions and then put all my effort into releasing all thoughts and physical sensations in the space between the contractions. Joel chanted along with me and that really kept me going. He was incredible, consistently reading my cues perfectly. One word or one gesture and he knew what to do—rub my back in a certain place with a certain amount of pressure, bring me water... I could really feel that the two of us together were bringing our baby into the world. And quite literally no one else was around. We were in a sleepy hospital on a Friday night and actually Valerie and the other midwives were in with another woman who was birthing her baby!

At a certain point the pain was very strong and I had a clear sense the prostaglandin gel should be removed. Joel managed to find a midwife who was doubtful that I could be progressing so fast but, after consulting Valerie, did agree to remove it.

My contractions continued to progress. At one point a midwife I'd never seen before strode into the room looking for a piece of equipment. She seemed totally unaware she was entering our space. Later she again strode in, this time probably to listen to our baby's heartbeat. Again, her energy did not feel 'in synch' to me. I felt very 'seated' in my power, like a lioness. I said emphatically to Joel: "Who is that? Tell her to leave." (I later learnt that he then took her aside and explained that I was a survivor of childhood sexual abuse and that I needed to feel very safe in my space. And she did improve.)

Eventually I remember making my way to the toilet. During my pregnancy I had the sense I would like to labour on the toilet because my pelvic floor muscles really could relax well there. This proved to be true. Through all the contractions my repetition of 'Om' continued, although the chanting eventually gave way to yelling! I would yell "Om!" as soon as the contraction began and continue all the way through it. The sounds that were coming out of me were incredible—they were deep, powerful sounds. I felt myself releasing on a very, very deep level what seemed like lifetimes of accumulated blockages. The process seemed to be freeing me from many of the wounds the abuse had left. I felt so much darkness that had previously taken up residence in my pelvic region being transmuted into light and being released through the sounds.

Unlike the abuse during which I 'left' my body, during the labour and birth I was fully present. As this moaning and purging was happening, I knew that a miraculous process was occurring. I was simultaneously reaching into the depths of where the abuse memories were stored in my physical body and into a depth of healing power which now seemed to interpenetrate the very same location. Quite literally the site of my childhood abuse was now the canal that my baby was soon to travel through. I tangibly felt that as the darkness was released through the sounds, my pelvis was opening, freeing everything up for my baby to move through. I was also aware even then that the impact of this experience would be far-reaching in my life and that I would be able to offer my child a much healthier mother. I felt grateful for this miraculous process.

At a certain point, I noticed myself very naturally starting to push at the end of each contraction. I had read that grunty pushes at the end of a contraction can help the cervix dilate. I had the sense I was getting close. I told my husband to get Valerie. She arrived and sat on the floor, Indian style, in front of me—and the toilet! She asked me if the sounds I was making were scaring me. I said "No". In fact, inside I felt very happy about the sounds as I knew what an incredible healing was taking place. I then mentally told the baby that everything was fine and not to be worried about the sounds, but my sense was that he or she was fine with it. From atop the toilet, I yelled and writhed and pushed my feet into Valerie's thighs during each contraction and then when the contraction was over I leaned forward and collapsed into her arms. This was an incredible part of the labour for me because I have never allowed myself to be mothered the way I allowed Valerie to mother me. I had felt engulfed by several women during my childhood and as an adult mostly avoided anything but loose hugs with other women. And here I was collapsing into Valerie's arms! This in itself was a whole other profound healing for me... I felt worthy of being mothered and I realised I wasn't defective in terms of allowing myself to be mothered when I was with a person I truly felt safe with.

I felt worthy of being mothered... I wasn't defective

Interestingly, at this point, my husband disappeared into the background for me. I specifically needed a woman to travel with me down this leg of the path, someone who had travelled this path before herself and accompanied other women down it. I later learnt Joel had taken a long-needed bathroom break!

I think Valerie noticed those grunty pushes I was doing at the end of the contractions and she asked to check my cervical dilation for the first time since labour had started. She also probably noticed me saying "I can't do it...," which is apparently a typical sign of being in transition. She checked and I was about 9cm dilated. I said "Thank God!" Valerie requested I move over to the bed, asking Ann and Joel to 'make it like a seat' since I was so reluctant to leave the toilet.

I laboured on all-fours for a while continuing to use movement and sound to cope with the pain of the contractions. I distinctly noticed my contractions become half as frequent. I understood I was in 'second stage' (fully dilated and pushing). My urge to push now took up much more of each contraction. It was so clear what my body was doing and so easy for me to follow along. At one point I spontaneously reached my hand into my vagina and I felt this mushiness which I knew to be the baby's head. I was so excited!

At some point I noticed the midwife was concerned that the baby's heartbeat was low. I remembered Ann explaining to us during an antenatal visit that sometimes when the birth is imminent the heartbeat will drop from head compression and that it was not dangerous. I was not concerned and said aloud: "It's just head compression".

Apparently, the baby's heartbeat continued to be low (at times 60 beats per minute). Now Valerie said "Bring the sound down lower out through your vagina" so I did. Then she said that we needed to have the baby born. By then I had flipped over onto my back. She asked me to pull up on my knees and do some forced pushes. Ann and Joel helped pull my legs up toward my chest. Of course, I didn't want to do this. I wanted to take my time and ease the baby out. I knew that both this position and forced pushing would be more likely to cause a tear and would decrease the oxygenation to the baby. Not wanting to do it and still wanting to do everything 'my way' I said "I can't". Valerie and Ann said firmly: "Do this for your baby." I pushed about twice and his head was out. One more push and his body swooshed out. The room was dark. Valerie held him up. He let out a cry. She said "The baby's fine" and immediately placed him on my belly. She said: "It was just head compression."

(It was only two years later, when consulting with another midwife, that I came to believe it to be a sensible practice for a midwife to 'want the baby born' when the heart rate has dropped for quite some time and is not resurging. My husband also told me that Ann said she would have done the same thing had our baby been born at home. I will never know for sure whether pushing him out before I felt ready was medically necessary. However, it was quite a profound moment for me. It was the moment that I did something I didn't want to do because the two midwives, whom I knew wanted to avoid all unnecessary interventions, both made it clear that it was for my baby. I felt Mother Nature was giving me a nudge to step out of the role of the individual 'Beth' and into the role of motherhood. I felt the birth of my motherhood was in that moment.)

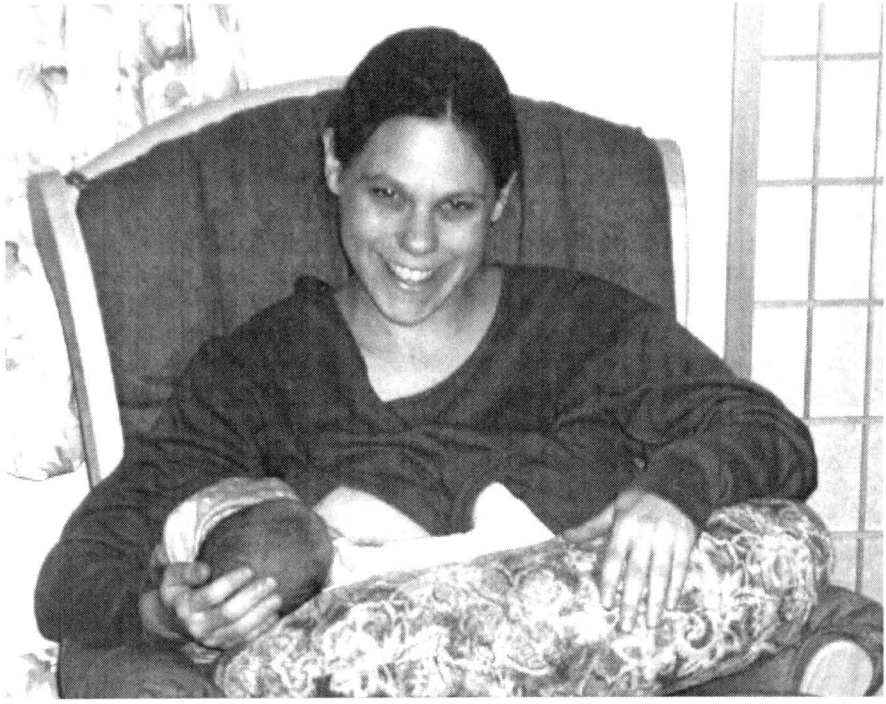

Comfortably breastfeeding

Our baby was so full and strong, not like the scrawny newborn I had expected. I rubbed his back and talked and talked and talked to him. It was so amazing to have skin-to-skin contact with him after having him inside me for so long. Since he was face down, I had no idea what he looked like or even if he was a boy or a girl. I just felt his body against mine and held him. Time stood still. After a while my husband suggested we cut the cord and see if we had a son or a daughter. (The placenta had already plopped right out after the baby was born). Then we discovered we had our Theodore and saw his beautiful face and beautiful body.

About 20 minutes after the birth, Ann helped me to breastfeed Theodore. He knew exactly what to do, which thrilled and amazed me and gave me confidence that breastfeeding would work out for us. Ann told us not to be surprised if he didn't feed as well the next few times, that in her experience babies often latch on very well right after the birth and then may need some help. I was so worried it somehow might not work out. I worried about whether Theodore's latch-on was correct. I leaked huge amounts of milk. I struggled with engorgement. I began to feel physically weak and emotionally overwhelmed five days after the birth. All of this while getting ready to move halfway across the country!

Luckily, when my friends asked how I was doing I honestly said: "Not well." We asked for help. Friends began coming to our home day and night helping pack, bringing food, feeding me and giving me emotional support. Their loving assistance touches me to this day.

By the time he was 12 days old, Theodore and I had got into a good rhythm with breastfeeding, my physical strength was gradually returning... and we were living in a new city! I struggled for several months adjusting to the changes in our lives—becoming a mother, leaving my previous employment, caring full-time for a new baby, living in a new city where I didn't know anyone, my husband working at a new job... And as I struggled with these changes, I would remember aspects of my birth experience and feel inspired and proud of my attainment. I also felt very proud and powerful that I was breastfeeding, that my body was nourishing my baby.

For the most part, I was able to tolerate the nearly constant physical closeness that my baby required. Occasionally, I felt overwhelmed at having him attached to my breast so often. During those times I sometimes imagined that the milk was flowing right out of my chest wall into him rather than coming out of my breast. I would concentrate on the sound and feeling of the milk gushing out of me and him gulping it down. This visualisation helped me forget about my breast and the emotional discomfort I was having with his suckling. I imagined myself giving him a person-to-person, life-generating transfusion.

I was amazed and grateful to find that most of the time I relished the physical closeness with Theodore. He wanted either to be held or breastfed day and night. Although it was exhausting to carry and breastfeed him constantly and I did not experience the kind of productivity I was used to in the working world, I was surprised at how often I felt a sense of fulfilment and accomplishment. I attribute this, in large part, to the mothering hormones released as a result of the frequent breastfeeding and nearly constant physical contact. I was surprised to find that my need to be with him was just as intense as his need to be with me.

By the time Theodore was 13 months old, I was able to appreciate how gradually, gently and naturally the process of him becoming independent and separating occurs. For example, in the early months he breastfed very, very often and was only content if we held him constantly. Then he began to crawl and sometimes preferred exploring to being held and even sometimes to breastfeeding! By 10 months he could walk and eat a little bit of food and could nap without being held, but he still relied very much on breastfeeding, being held and sleeping with us during the night. Then at 13 months he would breastfeed less frequently because he was really busy doing all his work and explorations. At that age, he would eat some solids but would rely mostly on breastmilk for his main source of nutrition. He slept with us and breastfed about one to three times during the night. Although at times he acted very independently, such as when he, on his own initiative, went upstairs when I was downstairs or darted off when we were in a shop, I could tell he very much still needed me to be there. I think that his confidence in knowing I was nearby helped him to feel safe to explore.

The key for me with breastfeeding a toddler is to make sure that I am comfortable emotionally and physically. As Theodore has grown, I have taken note of any aspects of our breastfeeding relationship that are uncomfortable for me and have sought to make adjustments as necessary. For example, when Theodore was under a year I enjoyed bathing with him and happily breastfed him in the bath. When he was about 18 months I began to breastfeed him in the bath and found that now with his bigger body and both of us undressed I didn't feel comfortable. As soon as I became aware of my discomfort, I stopped breastfeeding, got him involved in something else, and got myself dressed. In general, I noticed that when he breastfed with the intention of drinking milk, usually the milk flowed easily and his suck was comfortable for me. But sometimes when he 'hung out' on the breast I found it irritating. At these times he was usually willing to accept a snack, story or outing instead of breastfeeding. He often seemed to appreciate a substitution for breastfeeding because it actually better met his current need for attention, food, drink or interesting activity.

I would breastfeed him, but with awareness

When I wasn't keen on breastfeeding him but could tell he had a real need, I would breastfeed him then, but with awareness. Rather than sinking into feeling like a victim, I would remember that I'm his mother, a grown woman, choosing to meet my toddler son's needs. Then, as I watched him breastfeed and saw the relaxation and reprieve it brought him, and the relaxation it brought me, my choice was affirmed. Sometimes, when I was breastfeeding a bit reluctantly, it helped if I read while I did it. Reading helped me feel that I was giving something to myself as I breastfed Theodore. At other times I found that focusing fully on Theodore helped me shift into more positive feelings.

At other times, focusing fully on his feelings helped me shift into more positive feelings

Things changed for me when he was about 30 months. One night during that time, he asked to breastfeed. I was sleeping fairly deeply at the time and, and as he breastfed, I had the perception that someone was performing a sexual act on me. It turned out that Theodore's sucking on my breast was triggering a memory of my childhood abuse. Of course, Theodore was still his same little 2-year-old self and doing nothing unusual. But the size of his body (no longer a baby or a young toddler), his larger mouth and the difference in his suck, as well as it being during the night with me half-asleep all resembled the abuse too closely for my subconscious mind to differentiate. After that I gently and firmly discontinued night feeds, making it clear to him that although we wouldn't breastfeed at night, I'd still be there for him, responding to him. Whenever he requested the breast, I offered him a choice of water, a snuggle, or a snack. My husband offered to carry or rock him. We told him he could nurse again when it was light outside. Soon he often slept through the night.

As Theodore neared 3 years old, I began to resent his frequent requests for the breast throughout the day. Since, when he was younger, I had offered him the breast readily many, many times a day meeting his needs for food, drink, soothing, etc, he had come to think of breastfeeding as the thing to do whenever a need of almost any kind arose. I think this kind of thing is something many mothers (not only those who are abuse survivors) go through with breastfeeding children of his age. Theodore is quite verbal and I intuitively felt I was short-changing him if I didn't work with him to teach him other ways to meet his needs, verbalising his frustration or need for food or drink, seeking help in completing a project (rather than tossing the project aside in frustration and reflexively yelling, "Milk!"), asking for attention from me (rather than trying to get a 'piece' of me by breastfeeding).

> As he neared 3 years old I began to resent his frequent requests for the breast throughout the day

Also, I felt I was short-changing myself since, at this point, I did not enjoy feeding very much. Now, even when I'm fully awake while breastfeeding him, I often feel emotionally uncomfortable feeding such a big boy. My subconscious mind still 'reads' the breastfeeding as abuse and I usually want the feed to end as soon as possible. Two things have helped me during this stage. First, I have explained to him that he can breastfeed three specific times during the day: morning, after lunch, and after dinner. No longer do I have to respond to requests on a case-by-case basis, 20 times a day! I tell him clearly, "It's not time for milk" and offer other options instead. Second, I control the length of the breastfeeding session. Whenever I want it to end, I sing a specific song at a speed I determine. When the song is finished, Theodore stops feeding. He then often proudly says: "I stopped!"

Now, several months after his third birthday, Theodore continues to breastfeed three times a day but has indeed found other ways to meet his needs. For comfort he says "Cuddle me!" When hurt, he calls out woefully "I am hurt." He readily accepts snacks and drinks. I feel proud to see him growing up, yet continuing to express his needs so clearly and relationally.

What I've learnt...

This process of being attuned to my own experience and making adjustments as needed has been immensely healing for me, a survivor of childhood sexual abuse. When I was abused as a child, my own needs were not considered. I felt incapable and unworthy of asserting my needs.

Now, in relation to Theodore (now that he's 3—this didn't apply when he was a baby), I am able to assert my own needs as being important. Not more important than his needs, but also important. I have found, again and again, that we can find a solution that works to meet both our needs. Through our negotiations, not only am I teaching Theodore about the 'give and take' of healthy relationships, but I am learning about it myself.

I am teaching him about relationships and learning too

I now see that not only has breastfeeding been possible for me, a survivor of childhood sexual abuse, it has been immensely healing. My desire to have an empowering birth and fulfilling breastfeeding relationship has forced me to face emotional territory I would probably have otherwise avoided. One wound left by the abuse is an underlying sense of 'I can't do it. It's not even worth trying.' Birthing, breastfeeding and now the process of weaning Theodore have helped to replace this with a very real sense of capability and trust in myself. I am now confident that I can and will stand up for the well-being of myself and my child whenever necessary. I have also gained a heightened sensitivity to both myself and my son, which continues to serve us in our relationship as we both continue to grow and change.

Seeing what happens

Ashley Marshall

Harper's birth at home was sweeter than I could have dreamt it. I laboured easily and powerfully with loving support from my husband, doula and midwife. When Harper's bag of waters popped, birth energy rushed through me and soon his little head began to emerge. There was a slight case of dystocia and a tight umbilical cord but we were safe in the skilful hands of our midwife. Then, all of a sudden, there he was—pink, alert and beautiful.

The lotus birth was the right decision. It was the most beautiful beginning to following the culmination of pregnancy and the sense of loss that often ensues.

As I sat in awe of this perfect, wise being, I rubbed the creamy coating of vernix into his delicate skin and knew we had made the right decision to give him a lotus birth. It was the most blissful beginning to follow the culmination of pregnancy and the sense of loss that often ensues.

Lotus birth is the process of leaving the baby's placenta attached via the umbilical cord until it falls off of its own accord. Its purpose is both physiological and spiritual. Physiologically, the baby receives 43% of the blood left in maternal/placental circulation.

Ever wonder why cord blood banking has become so popular? It is known that cord blood—or blood left in the cord and placenta that hasn't made its way to the baby—is useful in helping to fight childhood leukemia later in that child's life. Why not stop denying a baby this vital blood and allow it to pass to the baby after birth instead? Also, the placenta is the baby's life preserver before breathing is established. As long as the cord remains intact and while it still pulsates the baby is being oxygenated.

Long after the cord stops pulsating and the physical transference is complete, the spiritual transference has only begun. This quiet time is when the baby's aura, or spiritual presence, is being realised. The placenta originated from the same cells as the baby and because of this bond they are a genetic identical of one another. A lotus birth allows for a respectful goodbye to the baby's womb mate.

How does a parent care for an intact placenta? It was surprisingly easy. After Harper's birth my husband and midwife placed it in a colander and rinsed all of the blood clots out. Then we rubbed it with sea salt and sprinkled it with lavender flowers.

Harper's placenta wore a cloth nappy just like he did and we changed it daily. We swaddled the 'placenta package' right along with him so we were free to pick him up, breastfeed and cuddle without the fear of tugging at his navel.

On the third day after his birth, Harper let go of his placenta. He was content and whole and ready to be free. We said goodbye to the organ that had nourished and protected our son for his first nine months but we will see it again when we plant it at Harper's first Blessing Way ceremony. In case you don't know, a Blessing Way ceremony is a Native American ritual used to mark significant life passages in one's life, frequently held to commemorate a birth, a marriage, a death or a woman's journey into motherhood. It is a more spiritual ceremony than the traditional American baby shower, where the focus is on showering the mother with gifts for the baby. A Blessing Way ceremony honours the mother and helps her draw upon her own inner resources that she will need later to give birth. My husband and I decided to offer our children a Blessing Way ceremony to celebrate their first year of life as well as my first year postpartum. We also planted their placentas at this time. (They were kept in the freezer up till then.)

Harper is our second child to be born at home, but our first lotus birth. We now know that we would never have another baby without giving them a lotus birth. It was three very mindful days that enabled us to remain in that warped sense of time that follows birth. We were surrounded only by love and close family while Harper made his earthly transition. There was plenty of time for lively celebration later that week but I will always be grateful for those precious days when Harper was lotus-born.

I will always be grateful for those precious days...

Ordinary, extraordinary adjustments...

Even if our situation seems entirely 'normal' and we make no unusual decisions when our babies are born, there is always something rather *extra*ordinary about childbirth. It's likely to take us by surprise whatever we do, whatever choices we make and whatever the outcomes. Here's hoping that your own experience will be extremely positive, in every possible way, and that you'll find ways of overcoming any potential or actual negatives. Life, whether it's ordinary or outrageously extraordinary is well worth adjusting to. Crossing the divide from single, carefree woman to mother inevitably sweeps us into another world, which visits to elderly relatives can never really reveal.

Experiencing a brave new world

Fiona Lucy Stoppard

My waters broke very, very early in the morning and then she wasn't born until after midnight. The labour was all that day—all morning, afternoon and evening—and she was born after midnight. So it was less than 24 hours. It was very slow for a long time. I phoned Michel and he said "Oh it's fine. It'll be all right. I'll come along later." I don't think I was having contractions then—only very slight ones. He came to see me, then he went home again. He was able to go backwards and forwards a little bit, although there was one point when he knew it was getting close and he said he'd stay.

I don't know what I can remember of the labour—it was just very hard work. A lot of resting. Very hard work. Completely closed off from the rest of the world. I remember asking David once to get me a mango and he went out and bought me a mango, which I didn't finish. It was actually too much to eat a mango because I had to concentrate. I went really deep, deep within. Quite spontaneously. But I don't see it as pain. After Amy's birth, I remember David answering a question from a friend: "How was it?" I can't remember his exact words but he said something like "Oh, God, it was hard." And I said, "It was not! It was wonderful!" I was being a bit defensive, but at the same time, I did feel like saying: "What are you talking about?" But he'd seen me go through all this seeming agony, making noises, faces, because some of my contractions were just—they just made me—it was extraordinary, the way I was bearing down, it was extraordinary. It was as if I was made of lead.

I suppose other people could have a lot of discomfort seeing and hearing the process of labour. It could be misinterpreted from the outside. I think it's something similar to lovemaking... being totally caught up in the moment, inside oneself, retreated from the outside world. And I remember that the next morning when I woke up I thought: "Oh, I'm here, back in the world again." I looked out of the window and people were doing normal, everyday things and I felt like saying: "Don't they realise what's just happened here?!"

Adjusting to a new reality

Sarah Hobart

When I was blessed a few years back with a baby boy, I had a vision. My life would go on much as before, only with a tiny baby keeping me company, smiling and gurgling as I went through the routines of daily living. That vision was almost immediately replaced by a reality where I barely maintained my sanity while struggling to meet the needs of one who, while adorable, was a tyrant. Any time of the day and especially at night I answered his clarion calls for "Milk, milk, milk, and step on it!" In those early weeks I was oblivious to everything but mastering this new role of motherhood.

It was then that I began to notice that not only had my world changed, but also I had changed. Namely, there seemed to be a lot more of me. 24 pounds more, to be exact. I told myself it was all in my breasts but that myth was dispelled after my husband pointed out that I was wearing maternity jeans. Embarrassed, I packed them away, and was left with a wardrobe of tracksuit bottoms and tight T-shirts.

I began to realise that not *only* had my world changed...

I told my doctor: "I think I have a glandular problem. All the other breast-feeding mothers are losing weight, but I hardly eat anything and I haven't lost an ounce!" She smiled gently and said: "If you burn more calories than you take in, you'll lose weight." She didn't believe me! I left her office in a huff, grumbling about the unfairness of it all. When did I, a new mother, ever have time for a meal? Most nights it was all I could do to grab a spoon and a pint of ice cream while my little one was nestled at my breast. I tried to ignore the growing problem of the larger me by avoiding full-length mirrors and clothes in general, but my new pounds fairly shouted for attention. They stood out in all sorts of awkward bulges, as if they'd been lobbed at me from some distance away and stuck fast. My ankles were thick and my feet were plump, my knees had a double chin and my midsection, well, let's just say I got tired of people asking me when my next baby was due. My upper torso was dominated by 'The Milk Factory', but the novelty of being well endowed quickly wore off. I wanted my old body back and was willing to try anything to get it. "I'll exercise," I declared. The local gym was advertising an aerobics class for new mothers. Babies were welcome. I signed up right away.

On class day, I struggled to get out of the house on time, lugging my son in a car seat that seemed to weigh 100 pounds. I couldn't find parking nearby, so I walked a few blocks with the car seat bashing into my shins. By the time I reached the gym, I was sweating profusely. Class had already started, led by a boyish woman with a body fat percentage of 3.0. She whipped the class through a routine of jumping, step climbing and marching that hurt every part of my body.

The other women moved smoothly through the programme while I focused on not looking like a fool, but I was always a step or three behind. Everyone was kind. I was glad, though, that my son slept through the entire pathetic performance. We went home and I weighed myself. I had lost a pound.

I went to my second class a few days later. This time I managed to keep up somewhat and even to throw some verve into my moves. As I leapt onto my step and threw my right foot out, I lost my balance and fell, knocking over the woman in front of me. Red-faced, I finished the class and went home to weigh myself. I had gained a pound.

I decided aerobics was not my 'thing'. Instead I bought a fancy jogging buggy, intending to zip around the block a few times a week with my baby riding in style. I had been an enthusiastic runner before my pregnancy, thinking nothing of knocking off two or three miles every other day. It wouldn't take long to fall back into my old habits. Everything went fine with my new programme until I came to my first hill and then I fell apart. It may as well have been Mount Rainier for all the gasping, grunting, and perspiring that went on—and that was just the first 20 yards. [Mount Rainier is a 14,410ft mountain in Washington State, USA.] I felt awkward not having my hands free and altogether discouraged with my outing. "My running days are over," I thought dispiritedly.

Right about then I decided to leave my fat where it was for a while and tackle another problem that had been bothering me—loneliness. My old friends didn't seem to understand my new life very well and sometimes blanched when I whipped out a breast to feed my son. I hadn't really got around to making new friends. So, despite my innate shyness, I dragged myself to a La Leche League meeting.

It was astonishing to see so many women brought together by a common interest, cheerfully breastfeeding their babies and discussing the changes motherhood had brought as if they actually relished their new lives. I really enjoyed my first meeting. I met someone there, a woman with a baby girl, who happened to live in my neighbourhood. Before long we had arranged to push our buggies around the lake a couple of times a week. She was such good company and we had so much in common that I really looked forward to these outings.

After a few weeks she suggested that we jog a little way each time we did our three-mile route, and it seemed like a good idea. The pace was never so strenuous that we couldn't keep talking. One day we were so engrossed in our subject (I think it was spit-up) that we jogged the whole three miles. It wasn't long after that that I put my sweatpants and my scales away.

My jogging and mothering buddy lives 600 miles away now... If I had any advice to give to other women in my shoes, it would be this: you are so much more than the sum of your parts. You're somebody's mother, for crying out loud! Life will never be the same, and neither will your body. It will be better.

Miraculously, you're nourishing a baby in the best way possible, using only your body, so despite its obvious flaws, strange bulges and odd sagging areas it's amazing. Focus instead on building and nurturing relationships with your child, your partner and especially other mothers. Have a 'tribe' with which to hang out, share stories, gripe, go to the park, exercise, talk parenting or any other subject... it'll make all the difference. The first year of new motherhood is tough. Establish a support network. You'll be glad you did when you discover how tough the second year is... and the third, fourth, fifth, etc. That would be my advice.

As for my own weight, the less I think about it, the happier I am! I don't look like a model but I feel great: fit, healthy and occasionally like Supermum. I didn't get my old body back... I got a more fun version with bigger boobs! I still exercise regularly and I'm still breastfeeding—my second baby now!

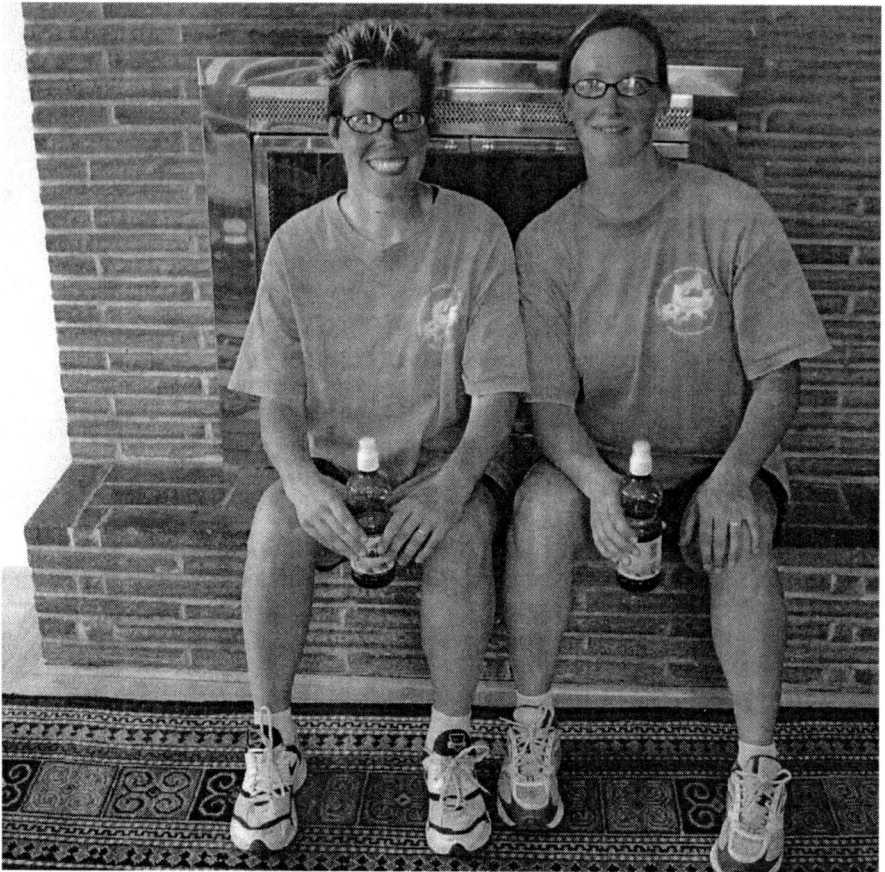

Sarah says: "That's me on the left with goofy hair, with my running buddy Ashly in Seattle, after a 'reunion run' of three miles."

Further reading

Books by Sylvie Donna:

- *Better Pregnancy, Better Birth*. Fresh Heart Publishing 2010.
  ISBN: 9781906619039.
- *Preparing for a Healthy Birth*. Fresh Heart Publishing 2010.
  ISBN: 9781906619053, 9781906619107 and 97819066015.
- *Optimal Birth: What, Why & How* (a book for midwives and other caregivers).
  Fresh Heart Publishing 2010. ISBN: 9781906619114.
- *Promoting Normal Birth: Research, Reflections & Guidelines* (for midwives).
  Fresh Heart Publishing 2010. ISBN: 9781906619060.

Books by Michel Odent:

- *Birth and Breastfeeding*. Clairview Books 2003 [first published in 1992].
  ISBN: 9781902636481.
- *The Caesarean*. Free Association Books 2004. ISBN: 9781853437182.
- *The Scientification of Love*. Free Association Books 1999. ISBN:
  9781853434761.

Other books to read while you're pregnant:

- *Pushed: The Painful Truth about Childbirth and Modern Maternity Care*
  by Jennifer Block. Da Capo Press 2008. ISBN: 9780738211664.
- *Birth Crisis* by Sheila Kitzinger. Routledge 2006. ISBN: 9780415372664.
- *Home Birth: A Practical Guide* by Nicky Wesson. Pinter & Martin 2006.
  ISBN: 9781905177066.
- *Silent Knife: Caesarean Prevention and Vaginal Birth After Caesarean* by
  Nancy Cohen and Lois Estner. Greenwood Press 1983.
  ISBN: 9780897890274.
- *Easy Exercises for Pregnancy* by Janet Balaskas and Anthea Sieveking.
  Frances Lincoln Publishers 1997. ISBN: 9780711210486.
- *Love is Not Enough: A Smart Woman's Guide to Money* by Merryn Somerset
  Webb. Harper Press 2008. ISBN: 9780007235193.
- *Breast is Best* by Penny Stanway. Pan Books 2005.
  ISBN: 9780330436304.
- *The Womanly Art of Breastfeeding* by Judy Torgus (ed.). Plume Books 2004.
  ISBN: 9780452285804.
- *Sleeping with Your Baby: A Parent's Guide to Cosleeping* by James
  McKenna. Platypus Media 2007. ISBN: 9781930775343.
- *Baby Wisdom* by Deborah Jackson. Hodder & Stoughton 2002.
  ISBN: 9780340793503.
- *The Attachment Parenting Book* by William and Martha Sears. Imported
  Little, Brown USA Titles 2001. ISBN: 9780316778091.

Who is Sylvie Donna?

Before she had children, Sylvie Donna worked in companies or taught English, mostly to working adults. She also trained teachers, or managed courses, departments—or a whole language centre in one case. She taught or organised courses for middle and top-level managers (as well as clerical or research staff) in Europe, North Africa, South Asia, South East Asia, the Middle East and the Far East. Her first book—*Teach Business English* (Cambridge University Press 2000)—is a synthesis of her experience in this field. Since having children, Sylvie has worked from home, writing and editing, or marking Master's assignments. She still does some teaching and lecturing at Durham University for MA, MSc, MBA and PhD students.

Sylvie started researching issues surrounding pregnancy and childbirth when she conceived her first child, which was also when she was finishing her own Master's degree. On the advice of a pregnancy book, she had started preparing a birth plan but she was surprised to find it was the cause of great discussion at each and every antenatal appointment. The implication to every objection seemed to be doubts about her ability to give birth. (Surely, she thought, her body should be capable of giving birth without too much intervention if it had managed to grow a baby in the first place?) In the end she decided to do even more research and she was reassured to find many studies which validated her choices. The only solution to the constant disagreements at antenatal appointments seemed to be to find another caregiver, which she then did—with some difficulty, it must be said. Perhaps it was because of her experience of working with managers and directors, that Sylvie found the confidence to challenge her caregivers when she disagreed with them!

After the birth (which went fine), Sylvie repeatedly met women who'd had bad experiences during their pregnancies or births and this led her to conclude that all her preparation—including her search for the right caregiver—had been helpful. Also, her experience of having the French obstetrician and male midwife Michel Odent attend her second birth made her realise that these women really were missing out on something quite wonderful: the instinctual experience of giving birth with what has been called a 'fetus ejection reflex'. (After exploring possibilities for birth while he was an obstetrician, Dr Odent became a researcher and homebirth midwife in London. His research has led him to conclude that birth is at its best when it is least disturbed.) Eventually, Sylvie did even more research, she collected lots of birth stories, some of which are in this book, wrote some more books—and had another baby!

Sylvie now attends many conferences on midwifery so as to continue to explore ways of helping women optimise their experience of birth and ways of making birth safer and more enjoyable for babies too. She is still very interested in finding out about *real* women's experiences, so please contact her when you've had your own baby to let her know how you got on.

Email: sylvie@freshheartpublishing.co.uk

Lightning Source UK Ltd.
Milton Keynes UK
17 May 2010

154281UK00001B/1/P